LESBIAN HEALTH

T0252807

LESBIAN HEALTH

What Are the Issues?

Edited by

Phyllis Noerager Stern, DNS, RN, FAAN, NAP

Indiana University School of Nursing
Indianapolis, Indiana

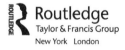
Routledge
Taylor & Francis Group
New York   London

USA	Publishing Office:	Taylor & Francis 1101 Vermont Ave., N.W., Suite 200 Washington, DC 20005-3521
	Distribution Office:	Taylor & Francis Inc. 1900 Frost Road, Suite 101 Bristol, PA 19007-1598
UK		Taylor & Francis Ltd. 4 John St. London WC1N 2ET

This edition published 2012 by Routledge:

Routledge
Taylor & Francis Group
711 Third Avenue
New York, NY 10017

Routledge
Taylor & Francis Group
2 Park Square, Milton Park
Abingdon, Oxon OX14 4RN

The papers in this book were originally published in the journal *Health Care for Women International,* Volume 13, Number 2, © 1992 Hemisphere Publishing Corporation, © 1993 Taylor & Francis.

LESBIAN HEALTH: What Are the Issues?

Copyright © 1992, 1993 Taylor & Francis. All rights reserved. Printed in the United States of America. Except as permitted under the United States Copyright Act of 1976, no part of this publication may be reproduced or distributed in any form or by any means, or stored in a database or retrieval system, without the prior written permission of the publisher.

This book was set in Times Roman by Taylor & Francis. The editors were Deborah Klenotic, Carolyn V. Ormes, and Miriam Gonzalez; the production supervisor was Peggy M. Rote; and the typesetter was Phoebe Ann Carter. Cover design by Michelle Fleitz.

A CIP catalog record for this book is available from the British Library.
♾ The paper in this publication meets the requirements of the ANSI Standard Z39.48-1984(Permanence of Paper)

Library of Congress Cataloging-in-Publication Data

Lesbian health: what are the issues? / edited by Phyllis Noerager
Stern.
    p. cm.
    "Originally published in the journal Health care for women
international, volume 13, number 2, 1992"—T.p. verso.
    Includes index.

    1. Lesbians—Medical are.   2. Lesbians—Health and hygiene.
3. Lesbians—Public opinion.   4. Medical personnel—Attitudes.
I. Stern, Phyllis Noerager.
    [DNLM: 1. Homosexuality.   2. Women's Health Services.   3. Women's
Health.   W1 HE299KG v.13 no. 2 1992 / WA 300 L623 1993]
RA564.87.L47   1993
362.1'08'6643—dc20
DNLM/DLC   93-3686
ISBN 1-56032-299-3   CIP

For Patsy and Karen

CONTENTS

CONTENTS

CONTRIBUTORS

JOYCE BAIN, RN, EdD
School of Nursing
University of Southern
  Mississippi
Hattiesburg, Mississippi
39406-5095

JULIE A. BUENTING, RNC,
  CNM, DNS
16 Hollybrook Road
Brockport, New York 14420

SHARON DEEVEY, RN, MS
College of Nursing
Ohio State University
Columbus, Ohio 43212

CAROL DONELAN, MA
Department of Comparative
  Literature
University of Massachusetts
Amherst, Massachusetts 01002

MICHELE ELIASON, PhD
College of Nursing
University of Iowa
Iowa City, Iowa 52242

SUSAN E. GENTRY, RN, BSN,
  MSN, ARNP
Division of Maternal-Fetal
  Medicine
College of Nursing
University of Florida
Gainesville, Florida 32611

LINDA HABER, RN, DNS, CS,
  PhD
Veterans Affairs Medical Center
Marion, Indiana 46953

JOANNE M. HALL, RN, MA,
  PhD
Department of Mental Health,
  Community, and
  Administrative Nursing
School of Nursing
University of California
San Francisco, California
94143-0608

JUDITH HOLLANDER, RN,
  MSN, CS
Veterans Affairs Medical Center
Fort Wayne, Indiana 46802

JANET W. KENNEY, RN, PhD
College of Nursing
Arizona State University
Tempe, Arizona 85281

VICKI A. LUCAS, RNC, PhD
Memorial Hospital Southwest
Houston, Texas

JILL RADFORD, MA
Rights of Women
52-54 Featherstone Street
London, EC1Y 8RT United
  Kingdom

CARLA RANDALL, MSN
Department of Nursing
Salish Kootenai Community
  College
Pablo, Montana 59855

M. MORAG ROBERTSON, MS,
  RNC, OGNP
Penquis Family Planning
Bangor, Maine 04401

PATRICIA E. STEVENS, RN,
  MA, PhD
Department of Mental Health,
  Community, and
  Administrative Nursing
School of Nursing
University of California
San Francisco, California
  94143-0608

DONNA T. TASH, RN, CNM
College of Nursing
Arizona State University
Tempe, Arizona 85281

SUSAN E. TRIPPET, RN, DSN
School of Nursing
University of Southern
  Mississippi
Hattiesburg, Mississippi
  39406-5095

LANA J. WALL, MSW
Alpatha Healing Center and
  Union Institute
Columbus, Ohio 43212

PREFACE

The year is 1990; the place, New Zealand; the event, the Fourth International Congress on Women's Health Issues. Five hundred women and a handful of men are feeling loving and strong and good about themselves.

Not quite all 500, as it turns out, for on the second day, a striking young woman mounts the platform and demands to know why we failed to include lesbian issues in the program. She tells us that almost one fourth of the audience call themselves lesbians and that they have come to the meeting expecting it to be relevant to their needs.

In the corridors, straight women, most of them academics, mutter, "Well, did anybody submit an abstract?" Because we all know the routine: you apply to present, and if the gods and the meeting judges smile on you, you become one of the chosen, and that most sacred of all academic documents, your curriculum vitae, gets another offering.

Coming out of the dining hall, I see the angry young woman. I ask her if any of her group have indeed applied to present a paper. Her disgusted retort is close to (but cleaned up for a family readership), "Cut the crap!" In my most placating tones I say something like, "Really, we've had papers about lesbians before; why nobody applied this time, I don't know." Not softening at all, she shoots back, "We're coming to the Council Board meeting; this isn't right." "Good," I say, "great!" Actually, I feel hurt, because I am being perfectly reasonable, but she isn't responding with reasonableness.

As the meeting of the Council Board of the organization that sponsors the biennial congresses comes to order, six women arrive together, take seats, and ask to speak. Their demeanor suggests challenge, aggressiveness. Members of the Board maintain their air of perfect reasonableness. A woman with an educated manner of speaking takes the lead and reads from a prepared document. She reproaches the Council for overlooking an important segment of womanhood in our congress. A Board member, perfect reasonableness waning, demands to know whether any of the lesbians applied to present a paper. At this point, Council Patron Afaf Meleis interjects that in her own work with minority groups she has learned that in gatherings such as the Congress, invitations must be extended to diverse groups; holding an open meeting is simply not enough.

Immediately the mood of the crowd changes. We all seem to know how affirmative action works—we need to let folks who are out of the mainstream know it is safe to participate. I for one feel like a fool.

Where is the sensitivity I claim to possess? I too work with minority populations. Why didn't I make the connection?

The lesbians read out their conditions. They demand that before the Fifth Congress in Denmark, a special issue of *Health Care for Women International* dealing with lesbians and their health must be released. I take pains to inform the petitioners that although *Health Care for Women International* may be the official journal of the Council, the readership extends far beyond that group, and that I as editor have sole control of its content. Having made my point, I agree to a special issue. (You bet I agree: a whole issue of a mainstream scientific periodical devoted to lesbian health sounds like a real breakthrough. The editor in me smells a scoop.)

And sure enough, the issue no sooner hits the streets in the summer of 1992 than it is sold out. We have to re-issue just to have copies available for the Copenhagen Congress in August.

In 1993 the publishers are hard put to keep up with requests for this special issue, and they make an important executive decision. They turn it into a book.

The journey from angry young woman to book is a real success story in a number of ways. For one who left San Francisco in 1980 thinking that all this gender-orientation nonsense was pretty well getting cleared up and accepted, editing the contents of this book is a real eye opener. Readers tell me it opens their eyes too. Unless your heart is of steel, there's stuff in here that will bring tears to your eyes. You will be outraged, as I am, at the prejudice, mistreatment, and downright ignorance held by even college-educated nurses! No wonder women are reluctant to come out as lesbians—it's dangerous out there.

The biggest success story for me is the response of lesbian readers. As Patricia Stevens writes in a letter to the editor of *Health Care for Women International*, "It is empowering for lesbians to hear that speaking up makes a difference." Making these matters public is about more than lesbians. It is about speaking up to make changes, and it is especially about extending our love and concern to all of our sisters.

Phyllis Noerager Stern

LESBIAN HEALTH CARE RESEARCH: A REVIEW OF THE LITERATURE FROM 1970 TO 1990

Patricia E. Stevens, RN, MA

Department of Mental Health, Community, and Administrative Nursing
School of Nursing, University of California, San Francisco

The author critically examines the research about health care providers' attitudes toward lesbians and the research about lesbians' experiences in health care encounters. Results of the review suggest that caregivers hold prejudiced views of lesbians and are generally condemnatory and ignorant about their lesbian clients. Lesbians frequently interpret caregivers' behaviors as hostile and rejecting and fear for their safety in health care interactions. Upon disclosure of their lesbian identity, many have been mistreated. Because of their negative experiences, they often delay seeking health care. Rather than conditions of respect and regard, lesbians report atmospheres of intimidation and humiliation, which encumber their interactions with health care providers. Tables outlining the study foci, samples, methods, and findings are provided. Ramifications of findings are discussed, implications for practice and policy are identified, and directions for future research about lesbian health care are suggested.

Reinforced by societal condemnation of lesbians, medical theories throughout this century have scapegoated and pathologized lesbians (Stevens & Hall, 1991). Until the late 1970s, lesbians were characterized by the medical profession as sick, dangerous, aggressive, tragically unhappy, deceitful, contagious, and self-destructive (Bergler, 1957; Caprio, 1954; Romm, 1965; Socarides, 1968; Wilbur, 1965; Wolff, 1971). Lesbians suffered exploitive treatments aimed at constraining their "homosexuality," including psychiatric confinement, electroshock treatment, genital mutilation, aversive therapy, psychosurgery, hormonal injection, psychoanalysis, and psychotropic chemotherapy (Abramson,

Patricia E. Stevens is a PhD candidate at the University of California, San Francisco.

1955; Adam, 1987; Council on Scientific Affairs, 1987; Doyle, 1967; Katz, 1976, 1983; Owensby, 1940; Robertiello, 1959; Seager, 1965). Their encounters with health care systems were fraught with the ideological construction of lesbianism as a sin, a crime, and a sickness.

The definition of lesbianism as disease at the turn of the century influenced a long history of scientific inquiry emphasizing etiology, diagnosis, and cure (Morin, 1977; Schwanberg, 1985, 1990; Watters, 1986). For 75 years lesbians were objectified in research designed to confirm the pathology of their condition. Such efforts isolated the phenomenon of being lesbian as an abnormality in need of explanation and assumed that lesbianism was an unhealthy disturbance that required prevention and treatment (Goodman, Lakey, Lashof, & Thorne, 1983; Lewes, 1988; Stevens & Hall, 1991).

This history underscores the vulnerable position lesbians occupy today as health care clients. Traditionally, lesbians' lives have been cloaked in secrecy and stigma. Society in the United States has persistently refused to acknowledge the existence of lesbians, their numbers in the population, and the variety of their life experiences (Wiesen-Cook, 1979). Lesbians' perspectives about health and their experiences in obtaining health care have also been ignored in scientific and clinical pursuits. An assertion made almost 20 years ago still rings true: "Male-dominated science has not taken women, including lesbians, seriously enough to engage in the necessary research on which the helping professions could adequately base their theory and practice" (Chafetz, Sampson, Beck, & West, 1974, p. 714).

By building a coherent body of knowledge about lesbian health care, we can facilitate the provision of accessible, comprehensive, and empathic care to lesbians. An important step in this process is to examine critically the investigations that have been done in this area. No thorough, scholarly review of the empirical literature about lesbians' experiences as health care clients has been done. My purpose in writing this article is to provide such a review. Implications for changes in practice and policy as well as directions for future research are also discussed.

The health sciences literature of the past 20 years was searched for any research related to lesbians' experiences with health care. The standard indexes to periodical literature and catalogs of doctoral dissertations were consulted. Additional studies were located through reference lists in published research and clinical articles about lesbians. A total of 28 studies were found, all conducted in the United States. Table 1 outlines 9 studies about health care providers' attitudes toward lesbian clients. Table 2 outlines 19 studies about lesbians' perceptions of their health care interactions. This second group of investigations used nonclinical samples of lesbians, unlike earlier medical "research" that

Table 1. Research on Health Care Providers' Attitudes Toward Lesbians

Study	Focus	Sample	Method	Findings
Levy (1978)	Psychology students' attitudes toward lesbians	San Diego; convenience; 106 students	Questionnaire	Lesbian clients were rated more negatively than heterosexual women clients with identical clinical presentations.
Implications: Knowledge of clients' lesbian identity alters health care providers' clinical assessments and subsequent diagnostic impressions.				
Liljestrand, Gerling, & Saliba (1978)	Sexual orientation and therapy outcomes	San Francisco; convenience; 24 clients, 16 therapists	Interview	More positive outcomes were reported when client and therapist were of the same gender and sexual orientation.
Implications: Gender and sexual orientation of health care providers can affect the potential for trust, empathy, openness, and respect in therapeutic encounters.				
Garfinkle & Morin (1978)	Health care providers' attitudes toward gays and lesbians	California; random; 40 female, 40 male psychologists	Questionnaire	Lesbian and gay clients were considered less healthy than heterosexual clients with identical clinical presentations. Males assessed lesbian clients more negatively than females.
Implications: Health care providers, particularly males, attribute poorer health to lesbian clients as a function of their own attitudes and values, believing health problems in lesbians to be more substantial and less amenable to change than similar problems in other clients.				

(Table continues on next page)

Table 1. Research on Health Care Providers' Attitudes Toward Lesbians (*Continued*)

Study	Focus	Sample	Method	Findings
White (1979)	Psychiatric nurses' attitudes toward lesbians	Midwest; convenience; 67 psychiatric nurses	Questionnaire	Greater religiosity was associated with greater negativity in attitudes toward lesbians. Nurses denied that their negative attitudes affected their clinical behaviors.

Implications: Although health care providers may believe that their negative perceptions do not interfere with the health care they deliver, their moralistic, condemnatory attitudes toward lesbians are probably detrimental.

Douglas, Kalman, & Kalman (1985)	RNs' and MDs' attitudes toward gays and lesbians	New York; convenience; 91 RNs, 37 MDs	Questionnaire	Homophobia scores of RNs and MDs were similar to those of the general public. Women were more homophobic than men.

Implications: Health care providers have many of the same prejudicial attitudes toward lesbians and gays that the larger society holds.

Mathews, Booth, Turner, & Kessler (1986)	MDs' attitudes toward gays and lesbians	San Diego; convenience; 1,009 MDs, 93% male	Questionnaire	23% were severely homophobic. Most homophobic: surgeons, gynecologists, and family practice MDs. 40% were uncomfortable with treating gays and lesbians. 30% opposed admitting gays and lesbians to medical schools. 40% would not refer clients to gay or lesbian colleagues.

Implications: A significant proportion of physicians hold very negative attitudes toward lesbians and are uncomfortable caring for them. Those specialties that display the most homophobia are the ones lesbians are most likely to come in contact with.

Study	Purpose	Sample/Setting	Method	Findings
Young (1988)	RNs' attitudes toward gays and lesbians	East coast; convenience; 22 RNs	Questionnaire	64% had negative attitudes toward gays and lesbians: pity, disgust, repulsion, unease, embarrassment, fear, and sorrow. 50% of RNs with these feelings stated that they had no desire to change.

Implications: Prejudicial feelings of such intensity are likely to interfere with nurses' ability to provide empathic and appropriate care to lesbian clients.

Study	Purpose	Sample/Setting	Method	Findings
Randall (1989)	Nursing educators' attitudes toward lesbians	Midwest; convenience; 100 nurses teaching in bachelor's of science in nursing (BSN) programs	Questionnaire	BSN educators' beliefs: Lesbianism is unnatural (52%), lesbians are disgusting (34%), lesbianism is immoral (23%), lesbians transmit acquired immune deficiency syndrome (AIDS) (20%), lesbianism is illegal (19%), lesbianism is a disease (17%), lesbians molest children (17%), lesbians are perverted (15%), and lesbians are unfit as RNs (8%). BSN educators' behaviors: Never discussed lesbian issues in the classroom (54%); were uncomfortable teaching or providing care to lesbians (28%).

Implications: Many nursing educators, whose behaviors and attitudes dramatically shape students' beliefs about clients and their comfort and skill in delivering nursing care, are ill informed about lesbians and hold negative attitudes toward them.

(Table continues on next page)

Table 1. Research on Health Care Providers' Attitudes Toward Lesbians (*Continued*)

Study	Focus	Sample	Method	Findings
Eliason & Randall (1991)	Nursing students' attitudes toward lesbians	Midwest; convenience; 120 female nursing students	Questionnaire	Nursing students' beliefs: lesbianism is unacceptable (50%), lesbians transmit AIDS (28%), and lesbianism is illegal (15%).

Implications: Many nursing students hold misconceptions and prejudicial attitudes about lesbians, which should be challenged in nursing curricula.

Table 2. Research on Lesbians' Health Care Experiences

Study	Focus	Sample	Method	Findings
Saghir & Robins (1973)	Lesbians' mental health	National; convenience; 57 lesbians, mean age of 31, all white and middle class	Structured interview	37% of lesbians were in therapy. One third of these evaluated therapy negatively, saying their therapists were prejudiced against lesbians.
Implications: Health care providers' (HCPs') attitudes and behaviors toward clients' sexual orientation affect lesbians' evaluations of therapeutic experiences.				
Chafetz, Sampson, Beck, & West (1974)	Lesbians' life experiences	Texas; snowball; 51 lesbians	Interview	Lesbians reported job discrimination, family and church rejection, public harassment, and forced psychiatric treatment. They were more likely to approach lesbian friends, instead of HCPs, in the event of illness.
Implications: Stigmatizing experiences affect help-seeking behaviors.				
Belote & Joesting (1976)	Lesbians' self-assessments	Florida; convenience; 82 lesbians, 16–44 years old, working class	Questionnaire	30% believed that HCPs discriminate against lesbians. 98% believed that they were mentally healthy as lesbians.
Implications: Although lesbians do not impute pathology to their sexual orientation, many believe that HCPs do.				

(Table continues on next page)

7

Table 2. Research on Lesbians' Health Care Experiences (*Continued*)

Study	Focus	Sample	Method	Findings
McGhee & Owen (1980)	Disclosure of sexual orientation to HCPs	San Francisco; convenience; 428 gay men, 157 lesbians	Questionnaire	73% had disclosed to HCP. 42% reported positive reactions when they disclosed. 31% of lesbians reported negative reactions. Many lesbians feared disapproval, insufficient diagnosis, and compromised treatment if they disclosed.

Implications: Lesbians have fears in approaching health care and risk negative reactions when they disclose their sexual orientation to HCPs.

Study	Focus	Sample	Method	Findings
Dardick & Grady (1980)	Lesbian and gay clients' disclosure of sexual orientation to HCPs	National; convenience; 491 gay men, 131 lesbians, 91% white, 22–41 years old, all middle class	Questionnaire	49% of lesbians disclosed to HCP or assumed HCP knew. Lesbians' perceptions of HCPs' feelings about gays affected disclosure rate. 27% reported overt hostility upon disclosure of lesbian identity. 18% of lesbians were dissatisfied with HCPs' prejudicial attitudes and heterosexual assumptions. HCPs' positivity toward disclosure improved client satisfaction and eased communication.

Implications: If lesbian clients perceive their HCPs to be nonjudgmental and open, they are willing to share the whole of their experiences and provide the information needed for delivery of the best possible health care. But previous negative interactions with HCPs can alienate lesbians from this process.

| Reagan (1981) | Lesbians' interactions with HCPs | Utah; convenience; 38 lesbians, mean age of 29, all white, middle and working classes | Questionnaire | 34% had disclosed to HCP. All were more comfortable and likely to disclose with female HCP. Most lesbians believed their health care would be of higher quality if they could safely disclose lesbian identity. Reported negative HCP reactions to disclosure were: anxiety, hostility, less likelihood of touch, mental health referral, excessive curiosity, and demeaning jokes. 25% delayed seeking health care because they feared disclosure consequences. |

Implications: Lesbians are very vigilant to verbal and nonverbal cues that a HCP feels uncomfortable, awkward, hostile, condemnatory, or accepting. Interactions with male HCPs can be especially discomforting.

| Johnson, Guenther, Laube, & Keettel (1981) | Lesbians' gynecological health care experiences | Midwest; convenience; 117 lesbians, mean age of 29, 95% white, middle class | Questionnaire | 40% feared the quality of their health care would be adversely affected if they became known as lesbians. 18% disclosed to HCP. 49% wanted to disclose to HCP if they could be safe. 91% preferred female HCP. 63% felt safer when accompanied by a friend. Many reported that HCPs' assumptions of heterosexuality reduced effective communication. |

(Table continues on next page)

9

Table 2. Research on Lesbians' Health Care Experiences (*Continued*)

Study	Focus	Sample	Method	Findings
				25% reported extremely poor experiences with obtaining gynecological care.

Implications: Lack of safety and openness in health care environments results in high rates of nondisclosure, fear, and negative health care experiences for lesbian clients.

Study	Focus	Sample	Method	Findings
Glascock (1981, 1983)	Lesbians' interactions with HCPs	New York; snowball; 27 lesbians, mean age of 39, all white and middle class	In-depth interview	50% avoided disclosing lesbian identity to HCPs. 50% feared sanctions and were seldom given opportunities to be open about themselves. Reported negative HCP behaviors were: hetero assumptions (85%), stereotyping (74%), ignorance (70%), denial of partner and social network (51%), attempts to cure lesbianism (48%), and breached confidence (22%). Some felt identifiable as lesbian even without a verbal disclosure. Trying to conceal lesbian identity caused problems. 55% hesitated to use the HC system.

Implications: HCPs' behaviors toward lesbian clients have implications for lesbians' access to and use of health care services.

Hume (1983)	Lesbians' disclosure decisions in health care situations	East coast; convenience; 63 lesbians	Questionnaire	Lesbians believed their health care would be of higher quality if they could safely disclose lesbian identity. Majority did not disclose; often delayed seeking health care; preferred lesbian HCPs; and were dissatisfied with HCPs' assumptions of heterosexuality, lack of knowledge about lesbian lives and health, and nonconfidentiality.

Implications: Many lesbians believe that unconstrained interpersonal disclosure in health care interactions would improve the quality of care offered to them and enhance their relationships with HCPs. They often delay seeking needed health care because of concerns about disclosure.

Olesker & Walsh (1984)	Lesbian mothers' experiences with obstetrical care	East coast; snowball; 9 lesbian mothers, mean age of 34, all white, middle and working classes	Structured interview	Most remained undisclosed when seeking prenatal care. Generally, lesbian mothers reported negative stereotyping by HCPs, exclusion of lesbian partners, or assumptions of heterosexuality.

Implications: Most HCPs assume that all women are heterosexual and direct their interactions accordingly. This can be particularly traumatic for lesbians and their partners who are seeking care for childbirth issues.

(Table continues on next page)

Table 2. Research on Lesbians' Health Care Experiences (*Continued*)

Study	Focus	Sample	Method	Findings
Smith, Johnson, & Guenther (1985)	Lesbians' gynecological health care experiences	National; convenience; 1,921 lesbians, 424 bisexual women, mean age of 28, 94% white, middle and working classes	Questionnaire	38% feared the quality of their health care would be adversely affected if they became known as lesbians.
				41% disclosed to gynecological HCP.
				36% wanted to disclose to HCP if they could be safe.
				21% believed gynecological health care improved with disclosure.
				93% preferred female HCP.
				50% felt safer when accompanied by a friend.
				Reported negative HCP reactions to disclosure were: embarrassment, rejection, voyeurism, mental health referral, coolness, and breached confidence.

Implications: Across the United States, lesbians believe that knowledge of their lesbian identity negatively affects the quality of health care they are offered. They worry for their safety in health care interactions.

Study	Focus	Sample	Method	Findings
Paroski (1987)	Health care concerns of lesbian and gay youth	New York; convenience; 89 gays, 32 lesbians, ages 14–17 years	Questionnaire and interview	Health care fears reported by lesbian and gay adolescents were: identification of sexual orientation, rough physical handling, rejection, HCP ignorance about lesbians and gays, and judgmental care. All preferred HCPs of the same gender and sexual orientation.
Implications: Lesbian and gay youth express multiple fears related to seeking health care, echoing many of the concerns of adult lesbians.				
Cochran & Mays (1988)	Disclosure to MDs by black lesbians	National; convenience; 529 lesbians, 65 bisexual women, mean age of 33, all black and middle class	Questionnaire	33% disclosed to HCP. 11% assumed HCP knew. Undisclosed lesbians felt alienated from the health care process and believed they received inappropriate care because of HCPs' assumptions of heterosexuality.
Implications: Black lesbians are reluctant to disclose their sexual orientation to HCPs, but nondisclosure has its own negative ramifications.				
Stevens & Hall (1988, 1990)	Lesbians' health care experiences	Midwest; snowball; 25 lesbians, mean age of 30, 92% white, middle and working classes	In-depth interview	72% reported negative HCP reactions to disclosure: ostracism, shock, pity, invasive questioning, fear, embarrassment, mistreatment of partners and friends, breached confidence, rough physical handling, derogatory comments, and pathological assumptions.

(Table continues on next page)

13

Table 2. Research on Lesbians' Health Care Experiences (*Continued*)

Study	Focus	Sample	Method	Findings
				Many felt identifiable as lesbians even without a verbal disclosure.
				Most were given few comfortable opportunities to disclose, even though they frequently wanted to.
				All believed some health care situations were too dangerous for disclosure.
				In unsafe health care environments they feared withdrawal of concern, inadequate care, and infliction of pain.
				They reported negative consequences of being undisclosed: invisibility, assumptions of heterosexuality, irrelevant health teaching, insensitive questioning, sexist remarks, improper treatment, and misdiagnosis.
				84% reported reluctance to seek health care.
				Reports of positive HCP behaviors included: open and inclusive language and approach, calm acknowledgment of lesbian identity, support, regard, respect, welcoming of their partners and friends.
				They preferred female HCP.

Implications: Lesbians often do not feel comfortable seeking health care, experience nonempathic responses when they do, and even feel at risk of harm in some health care situations.

Bradford & Ryan (1988)	Lesbian's health concerns & health care needs	National; convenience; 1,925 lesbians, mean age of 33, 88% white, 6% black, 4% latina, all middle class	Questionnaire	Reported problems in obtaining health care were: assumption of heterosexuality, lack of safety for disclosure, HCPs do not listen and encourage open communication, lack of mutual decision making, forced birth control, and rough physical handling. Some feared the quality of their health care would be adversely affected if they became known as lesbians. Most common reasons for not seeking needed health care were lack of financial resources and distrust of HCPs. The majority preferred female HCPs.

Implications: If assumption of heterosexuality is pervasive, lesbian clients are invisible. This makes it difficult for them to fully discuss their health concerns.

Saunders, Tupac, & MacCulloch (1988)	Lesbians' general life experiences	Los Angeles; convenience; 1,000 lesbians, mean age of 36, 91% white, all middle class	Questionnaire	Many were more likely to seek help for a health problem from lesbian friends rather than HCPs. They sought help from HCPs through referrals from lesbian friends. Some feared disapproval from HCPs and subsequent decreased quality of care.

Implications: Connections with lesbian social networks are very important in lesbians' help-seeking behaviors.

(Table continues on next page)

Table 2. Research on Lesbians' Health Care Experiences (Continued)

Study	Focus	Sample	Method	Findings
Harvey, Carr, & Bernheine (1989)	Obstetrical experiences of lesbian mothers	National; convenience; 35 lesbians, mean age of 34, 94% white, all middle class	Questionnaire	91% disclosed to their obstetrical HCP. 79% reported that this HCP was supportive. 10% reported that they were refused obstetrical health care because they were lesbian. 50% rated HCPs in general as ill informed about lesbians and uncomfortable in providing care to lesbians.

Implications: Many lesbians are generally critical of HCPs' knowledge of and sensitivity to lesbian's health care concerns.

Study	Focus	Sample	Method	Findings
Zeidenstein (1990)	Lesbians' disclosure experiences in ob/gyn health care	East coast; snowball; 20 lesbians, 31–49 years old, 90% white, all middle class	Structured interview	50% disclosed to HCP to dispel assumptions of heterosexuality. 25% worried about confidentiality. Most were given few comforatable opportunities to disclose. Some disclosed to HCP in response to harassment. Reported consequences of nondisclosure were: inaccurate health teaching and misdiagnosis. 50% reported delaying health care because of fears about mistreatment by HCPs. 50% felt safer in HC when accompanied by a partner.

Implications: Lesbians perceive few positive opportunities for disclosure and have significant fears about their safety in health care encounters.

| Deevey (1990) | Health behaviors of older lesbians | National; convenience; 78 lesbians, over age 50, 99% white, all middle class | Questionnaire | 80% reported discrimination because of lesbian identity. Majority mistrusted mainstream health care. Many were offended by labels and did not wish to disclose in health care situations. |

Implications: Lesbians' desires and comfort related to disclosure in health care situations vary according to age, general comfort with disclosure, safety of the environment, and previous experiences with HCPs.

based conclusions about lesbians on case studies of women incarcerated in prisons and mental hospitals (Stevens & Hall, 1991).

It is significant that these 28 studies were undertaken. Their existence attests to the fact that some nurses, psychologists, public health administrators, social workers, and physicians have recognized that lesbians face significant difficulties in health care interactions. Moreover, these investigators have had the courage to speak publicly. Although the political climate in these disciplines is changing, many scholars have been deterred from researching and writing about lesbian topics because their association with lesbian populations posed risks of personal stigmatization.

HEALTH CARE PROVIDERS' ATTITUDES TOWARD LESBIANS

From the findings of the nine studies that specifically explored health care providers' attitudes toward lesbians, it is clear that prejudice is alive and well in present-day clinical practice and health care provider education (see Table 1). This survey evidence suggests that lesbianism was still considered an affliction by many health care providers (Randall, 1989; White, 1979; Young, 1988). As a result, they made pathological assumptions, conceptualizing lesbianism as an illness in and of itself or seeing it as a condition to which a wide variety of health problems can be attributed.

Clinicians imputed greater psychological maladjustment to lesbian clients than to heterosexual controls with identical clinical case presentations (Garfinkle & Morin, 1978; Levy, 1978). Significant numbers of physicians and nurses were uncomfortable providing care for lesbian clients, regularly refused service to women who were lesbian, were unwilling to discuss lesbian issues in the classroom, and believed that lesbians should not be allowed to become health care providers (Harvey, Carr, & Bernheine, 1989; Mathews, Booth, Turner, & Kessler, 1986; Randall, 1989). Many inappropriately associated high rates of human immunodeficiency virus infection and transmission with lesbian clients, presumably because they were unable to distinguish lesbians from gay men (Eliason & Randall, 1991; Olesker & Walsh, 1984; Randall, 1989). Damaging stereotypes that are widespread in the general public were also apparent in the way nurses and doctors thought about lesbians; for example, lesbians were viewed as "unnatural," "disgusting," "immoral," "perverted," "criminal" (Douglas, Kalman, & Kalman, 1985; Eliason & Randall, 1991; Mathews et al., 1986; Randall, 1989). The emotions evoked by their interactions with lesbian clients included pity, disgust, repulsion, unease, embarrassment, fear, and sorrow (Randall, 1989; Young, 1988).

Because all of the studies in this group were based on questionnaire methods, the social desirability factor must not be ignored. Were providers giving answers they believed researchers wanted to hear? Is it possible that their attitudes toward lesbians were even more negative? Also, because these were, for the most part, convenience samples, we do not know the attitudes of providers who declined to participate. Were they likely to have more or less affinity toward lesbian clients?

Other researchers have shown that prejudices about race, gender, class, and nationality prompted differences in diagnosis and treatment that were not attributable to variation in the conditions of the clients (Anderson, 1985; Fisher & Groce, 1985; Hurst & Zambrana, 1980; Jonas, 1974; La Fargue, 1972; Roth, 1986; Shaw, 1971; Todd, 1989; Waitzkin, 1983; Waitzkin & Waterman, 1974; Zola, 1972). Although some providers protested that their moral biases and social judgments did not affect the health care they provided to lesbians (White, 1979), it is more likely that daily activities with clients reflect and reinforce health care providers' prejudices.

LESBIANS' HEALTH CARE EXPERIENCES

Findings of the 19 studies of lesbians' perspectives about health care indicate that anti-lesbian ideas and sentiments are conspicuous in the behaviors of health care providers (see Table 2). Several trends in the research findings did not vary appreciably over the last two decades or on the basis of regionality. For example, lesbians believed health care providers were generally condemnatory toward and ignorant about them. They frequently interpreted health care provider behaviors as hostile and rejecting and feared for their safety in health care interactions. Upon disclosure of their lesbian identity, they experienced many kinds of mistreatment. Because of their negative experiences, they were often reluctant to seek health care. Rather than conditions of respect and regard, lesbians reported atmospheres of intimidation and humiliation, which encumbered their interactions with health care providers. These claims are detailed in the following sections.

Ignorance and Antipathy

The studies were nearly unanimous in showing that health care providers' heterosexual assumptions were a major hindrance to effective therapeutic communication. Results revealed that providers usually assumed that their female clients were heterosexual, had male sexual partners, and performed within normative social roles as wives and mothers in traditional family units. Very rarely were there comfortable opportunities for lesbian clients to let providers know that they were not heterosexual. According to lesbian clients, such conditions made them feel invisible and led providers to misdiagnose conditions, provide inadequate treatment, offer irrelevant health teaching, lecture about birth control, ask insensitive and biased questions, make sexist remarks, and alienate lesbians from the entire health care process (Bradford & Ryan, 1988; Cochran & Mays, 1988; Glascock, 1981, 1983; Johnson, Guenther, Laube, & Keettel, 1981; Olesker & Walsh, 1984; Stevens & Hall, 1990; Zeidenstein, 1990). Such assumptions also robbed providers of access to practical knowledge about lesbian life experiences, health concerns, community resources, and support networks.

In addition to the problem of ignorance about lesbian existence, lesbians reported that they were pathologized when they *were* known to be lesbian. Their presenting problems were ignored while their lesbianism became the object of concern. Some women were inappropriately referred to mental health professionals (Belote & Joesting, 1976; Chafetz et al., 1974; Glascock, 1981; Reagan, 1981; Smith, Johnson, & Guenther, 1985; Stevens & Hall, 1988). A few even reported that a male physician attempted to "cure" their lesbianism by making sexual advances toward them (Bell & Weinberg, 1978; Glascock, 1983). Such abuse and the disease attributions proved detrimental to lesbians' confidence in the health care system and their sense that health care providers were knowledgeable and concerned about their health and well-being.

Lesbians generally described health care providers as misinformed and prejudicial (Belote & Joesting, 1976; Dardick & Grady, 1980; Johnson et al., 1981; Olesker & Walsh, 1984; Paroski, 1987; Reagan, 1981; Saghir & Robins, 1973). They reported that they spent an exorbitant amount of their health care time educating providers about lesbianism and dissuading them from stereotypes. One researcher concluded, "Stereotyped misconceptions leave professionals with homophobic fears, inaccurate assumptions, unanswered questions, and misinterpreted symptoms" (Reagan, 1981, p. 25).

Significant numbers in several of the investigations believed that care was compromised because of their lesbianism. As a result, they often characterized health care situations as dangerous (Bradford & Ryan, 1988; Glascock, 1981; Johnson et al., 1981; McGhee & Owen, 1980; Paroski, 1987; Saunders, Tupac, & MacCulloch, 1988; Smith et al., 1985; Stevens & Hall, 1988, 1990). They feared they might be harmed in health care interactions if they became known as lesbians; some only felt safe when accompanied by a partner or friend who could act as a witness and advocate (Johnson et al., 1981; Olesker & Walsh, 1984;

Smith et al., 1985; Stevens & Hall, 1988; Zeidenstein, 1990). There were indications that some health care contexts were perceived as more hazardous, such as emergency services, inpatient hospital care, long-term care, surgery, and any other circumstances wherein lesbians had little chance to select who might be caring for them (Stevens & Hall, 1990).

According to this group of studies, lesbian clients tended to be very vigilant for behavioral and verbal cues from health care providers that conveyed their openness toward or discomfort with lesbians. One researcher summed it up: "Because lesbians . . . negotiate their daily lives in environments that range from hostile to friendly, they are acutely aware of subtleties in language and manner that suggest danger or safety" (Deevey, 1990, p. 37).

Disclosure of Lesbian Identity

Such sensitivity to the behavior of others influenced lesbians' decisions regarding disclosure in health care encounters. Empirically based wisdom suggests that decision making regarding disclosure of lesbian identity is more complicated than the metaphor of being in or out of the closet might suggest (Brooks, 1981; Schneider & Conrad, 1986; Stevens & Hall, 1988; Wells & Kline, 1987). The degree of lesbians' openness about themselves is guided by the contingencies of particular interactions. In each context they must imaginatively construct the anticipated responses of others while balancing personal vulnerability and available resources, in an attempt to avoid social rejection, humiliation, restriction, or attack.

Many lesbians believed that the quality of their relationships with providers would improve if they could feel free and safe to acknowledge their identities as whole persons and share the details of their social, emotional, and sexual lives when appropriate (Dardick & Grady, 1980; Hume, 1983; Johnson et al., 1981; Reagan, 1981; Smith et al., 1985; Stevens & Hall, 1988). However, efforts at disclosing lesbian identity in health care encounters evoked a wide array of reactions on the part of providers, ranging from embarrassment to overt hostility. Reported responses from health care providers included fear, ostracism, refusal to treat, cool detachment, shock, pity, voyeuristic curiosity, demeaning jokes, avoidance of physical contact, insults to them and their lesbian partners and friends, invasions of privacy, rough physical handling, and breaches of confidentiality (Dardick & Grady, 1980; Glascock, 1981, 1983; Harvey et al., 1989; Hume, 1983; McGhee & Owen, 1980; Paroski, 1987; Reagan, 1981; Smith et al., 1985; Stevens & Hall, 1988, 1990).

Because of negative ramifications, many women did not feel free to disclose that they were lesbians in health care contexts, even when they would have preferred to do so (Cochran & Mays, 1988; Dardick & Grady, 1980; Glascock, 1981; Hume, 1983; Johnson et al., 1981; Olesker & Walsh, 1984; Reagan, 1981; Smith et al., 1985; Stevens & Hall, 1990; Zeidenstein, 1990). Because of nondisclosure, they were subjected to providers' heterosexual assumptions and subsequently paid the price of alienation, feeling like outsiders or pariahs. While withholding information about themselves they risked being provoked into rash, unplanned disclosures (Gonsiorek, 1988). Sometimes the disclosures reported by lesbian research participants could not be characterized as voluntary. Several women described health care circumstances in which they felt forced to disclose or did so impulsively in response to harassment (Stevens & Hall, 1988; Zeidenstein, 1990).

A tremendous loss of time, energy, self-worth, and authenticity can be exacted by the vigilant monitoring process involved in nondisclosure (Erlich, 1981; Hetrick & Martin, 1987; Jandt & Darsey, 1981). Jones et al. (1984) suggested, "A person who exerts tremendous effort to keep some personal information from public attention may continually focus on the stigmatizing implications of this secret knowledge, and consequently maintain its salience in self-definition" (p. 129). Nevertheless, nondisclosure in unsafe environments is a survival strategy (Nungesser, 1983). The decision to try to avoid disclosure arises under conditions of normative proscription. Even among women who have not had personal experiences with discrimination when they disclosed their lesbianism to health care providers, the negative experiences of other lesbians and the stories that circulate about such incidents act as strong deterrents (Stevens & Hall, 1990).

Verbal disclosure of lesbian identity is an irrevocable revelation. However, it is not the only means by which lesbians become known in health care situations. Many women believed that their lesbianism was readily apparent by their physical appearance, their manner, the content of their conversation, their associates, and/or their living arrangements (Deevey, 1990; Glascock, 1983; Moses, 1978; Stevens & Hall, 1988; Zeidenstein, 1990). For some women, information about their lesbian identity was not perceived as being under their personal control. For others who believed they could conceal their lesbian identity, comprehensive management of that information involved not only keeping silent about being lesbian, but also being vigilant about the intimate details of who they were, how they acted, how they looked, what they said, who they were with, and where they went. Such a task is extremely complex and is not paralleled in the experiences of nonlesbian women.

Research has indicated, moreover, that lesbians can be victims of discrimination whether or not they verbally disclose their lesbian identity. The patterns of civil liberties violations and abuse are similar whether sexual orientation is assumed, based on rumor and opinion, or known, based on public record or verbal acknowledgment (Goodman et al., 1983; Liljestrand, Petersen, & Zellers, 1978; Schneider, 1982).

Delayed Help Seeking

Many of the investigators found that lesbians delayed seeking health care because of their fears and poor health care experiences (Bradford & Ryan, 1988; Chafetz et al., 1974; Deevey, 1990; Glascock, 1981; Hume, 1983; Reagan, 1981; Stevens & Hall, 1988; Zeidenstein, 1990). In some cases they were more likely to seek help from lesbian friends rather than from health care providers (Chafetz et al., 1974; Saunders et al., 1988). When lesbian clients perceived health care encounters as inadequate and providers as rejecting, insensitive, or frightening, they were unlikely to return to those settings, which limited their health care options. Institutional structures and policies also inhibited lesbians' access to health care services, including those that denied visitation and involvement of lesbians' significant others, located women's preventive health services exclusively in birth control and obstetrical clinics, ignored outreach to lesbian communities, and inhibited lesbian nurses and physicians from coming out. Insurmountable economic barriers to care were also identified (Bradford & Ryan, 1988; Glascock, 1981; Stevens & Hall, 1988). Financial access to care is particularly problematic for women who live outside heterosexually constructed nuclear families, unattached to adult male incomes. Women workers in the United States are paid inequitable wages, receive less extensive health benefits, and are more likely to be without health coverage of any kind (Stevens, in press). Lesbians also cannot claim partners or the children they co-parent as dependents on health insurance policies.

Lesbians described conditions that would increase their comfort in seeking health care. For instance, when asked, lesbian clients expressed an overwhelming preference for female health care providers, especially if they were lesbian (Bradford & Ryan, 1988; Glascock, 1981; Hume, 1983; Johnson et al., 1981; Liljestrand, Gerling, & Saliba, 1978; Olesker & Walsh, 1984; Paroski, 1987; Reagan, 1981; Smith et al., 1985; Stevens & Hall, 1988). With women they felt more comfortable, perceived more kindness and openness, and believed that they were less vulnerable to harm. Because so many lesbians preferred being accompanied by a significant other, receptivity toward lesbian partners and friends was also evaluated very positively (Dardick & Grady, 1980; Johnson et al., 1981; Reagan, 1981; Smith et al., 1985; Stevens & Hall, 1988).

The relational qualities lesbians identified as important in health care encounters were trust, openness, acceptance, and understanding (Johnson et al., 1981; McGhee & Owen, 1980; Olesker & Walsh, 1984). They suggested that one of the fundamental ways health care providers could demonstrate commitment to these relational ideals was through inclusive language and behaviors, whereby they did not assume heterosexuality (Dardick & Grady, 1980; Harvey et al., 1989; Johnson et al., 1981; Olesker & Walsh, 1984; Reagan, 1981; Smith et al., 1985; Stevens & Hall, 1988; Zeidenstein, 1990). Lesbian participants were also clear that they did not want providers to blindly and naively enter into health care interactions with them. Instead they believed that nurses, physicians, and other providers were accountable for acknowledging their prejudices and working to eliminate them. They expected providers to be well informed about lesbian life and knowledgeable about lesbian health, so that they could provide comprehensive services and make appropriate recommendations. They suggested that health care providers improve their practices by becoming familiar with lesbian health research, reading from the abundance of lesbian literature, and consulting lesbian community resources.

DISCUSSION

This review of the empirical literature on lesbians' health care experiences suggests that deeply entrenched prejudicial meanings about lesbian health remain influential in the education of health care providers, the quality of health care they deliver, their comfort in interacting with clients, and the institutional policies under which they work. Knowledgeable, empathic, and fully accessible care cannot coexist with such conditions. The present findings indicate that many lesbians interpret health care interactions as abusive and perceive high-quality, safe health services to be unavailable to them. Such findings are of serious concern and call for immediate radical changes on the part of educators, practitioners, administrators, and policymakers.

The 20 years of research reviewed herein gives evidence that we must transform not only individual behaviors, but also systems of care delivery and systems of education. Everyone and every place that provides care to women provides care to lesbians. Individual providers must take note of their own knowledge, attitudes, and behaviors and also think on an institutional level and mobilize collectively to make changes. We are accountable for the structures in which we work, the actions of co-workers, and the public stands taken by our professional organizations.

Do we insist on policies that are inclusive of lesbians? Do we object vigorously to atmospheres that threaten or badger clients? Do we call colleagues on prejudicial behaviors? Do we persevere in integrating lesbian content into the entire curricula of women's health, family health, and adolescent health?

Because as providers of health care we are in a more powerful position than recipients, we carry the responsibility for creating openness and receptivity, rather than expecting lesbian clients to overcome myriad barriers to get taken care of properly. If we create environments and pursue verbal and written assessment methods that do not presume the circumstances of clients' relational and sexual lives, we can avoid premature foreclosure of communication. If we calmly, knowledgeably, and supportively approach our clients, accepting whatever they choose to share about themselves with respect and regard, we can begin to ensure safety and comfort.

There are also implications for research and knowledge development. An unsettling observation derived from this review is that extant research about lesbian health care overwhelmingly reflects the experiences of white, middle-class, well-educated lesbians, aged 20 to 40. Even these women, many of whom had health insurance and access to private care, were reluctant to seek mainstream health services and reported very negative experiences with physicians, nurses, and others. What about lesbians who must receive care from public-sector facilities because they are poor and/or uninsured? How satisfactory and accessible is their health care? What are the experiences of lesbians of color, who must contend with racism as well? Gender, economic, and racial hierarchies operate simultaneously with enduring societal values on traditional heterosexuality to intimately affect the health care experiences of lesbians. We need to find out the details of how this occurs, so that we can improve our practices. Appreciating the complexity and diversity of women's lives, we must expand the boundaries of our populations of interest and take deliberate actions to facilitate the participation of women who have historically been excluded from research (Hall & Stevens, 1991).

Not only are there segments of lesbian populations about whom we know very little, but the studies we do have are rather limited in scope. They are most instructive about disclosure of lesbian identity in health care situations, lesbians' experiences in routine visits to doctors' offices, and attitudes toward lesbians that providers are willing to admit to on paper-and-pencil tests. Major knowledge deficits remain regarding lesbians' access to health care services, the ways they seek help for health problems, how they conceptualize their health, their experiences with health care providers across a full range of health care contexts, and how health care providers' attitudes correspond with their actual behaviors toward lesbian clients.

This research review raises several questions that may be fertile ground for future research. How is disclosure associated with the whole interactional and structural context of health care? How can institutions and individual providers facilitate lesbians' use of services? What ramifications does the profit-based organization of the U.S. health care system and health insurance industry have for lesbian consumers? Are there links between the interactional circumstances of lesbians' encounters with health care providers and their health outcomes? How do the processes of encounters involving emergency health problems differ from those of a more routine nature? What are the health care issues for lesbians with chronic conditions who must make repeated contacts with health care systems over long periods? What are the roles of lesbian communities and friendship networks in lesbians' health promotion and maintenance? What are lesbians' most pertinent health concerns? It would also be very helpful to have more empirical information about lesbians' experiences with various health care personnel, including hospital staff nurses, nurse practitioners, medical specialists, mental health professionals, and nonallopathic practitioners. Lesbians' encounters in different kinds of facilities, such as emergency rooms, health maintenance organizations, public hospitals, and substance abuse treatment centers, are also pertinent.

Methodologically, there is room for more creativity and a need for more adequate financial support of lesbian health research. The present findings suggest that we need to explore more direct ways of capturing the effects of attitude on the care clinicians deliver; the education offered in schools of nursing, medicine, and other health professions; and the policies of health care institutions. We need to examine which research questions call for qualitative methods in natural settings versus mailed surveys or other quantitative methods. Are there innovative designs that could be effective in exploring this relatively unknown area of women's health care? Do good models of health care delivery for lesbians exist, on which we might base demonstration projects? Most of the studies in this review were accomplished on shoestring budgets or were projects in fulfillment of a master's or doctoral degree. We need to find sources of institutional and municipal funding and extramural grants that can be tapped to support more and varied studies, cumulative programs of research, and large-scale team efforts.

Innovative sampling methods are also called for. How can we reach more diverse segments of the lesbian population, and how can we improve our sampling strategies, given the constraints involved in studying a largely hidden and historically invisible population such as lesbians?

Samples must be drawn from a universe whose limits, units, and locales are largely unknown. Conventional mathematical sampling techniques that strive for random composition, representativeness, and/or structured comparison groups are simply not scientifically feasible in studying this population.

Some of the studies reviewed herein were unpublished or available only through nonprofit organizations, decreasing their potential impact. Others appeared in scholarly journals. None are available in the lay or government press. We must try to determine the most effective ways of disseminating results of research about lesbian health to lesbian populations as well as to a wide range of health care providers and policymakers, so that we can facilitate much-needed changes. Research is a very powerful political tool. A sound knowledge base can empower lesbian clients and help us make health care more accessible to and appropriate for lesbian populations.

REFERENCES

Abramson, H. A. (1955). Lysergic acid diethylamide (LSD-25): As an adjunct to psychotherapy with elimination of fear of homosexuality. *Journal of Psychology, 39,* 127–155.

Adam, B. D. (1987). *The rise of the gay and lesbian movement.* Boston: Twayne.

Anderson, J. M. (1985). Perspectives on the health of immigrant women: A feminist analysis. *Advances in Nursing Science, 8*(1), 61–76.

Bell, A. P., & Weinberg, M. S. (1978). *Homosexualities: A study of diversity among men and women.* New York: Simon & Schuster.

Belote, D., & Joesting, J. (1976). Demographic and self report characteristics of lesbians. *Psychological Reports, 39,* 621–622.

Bergler, E. (1957). *Homosexuality: Disease or a way of life?* New York: Hill & Wang.

Bradford, J., & Ryan, C. (1988). *The national lesbian health care survey.* Washington, DC: National Lesbian and Gay Health Foundation.

Brooks, V. (1981). *Minority stress and lesbian women.* Lexington, MA: D. C. Heath.

Caprio, F. S. (1954). *Female homosexuality: A psychodynamic study of lesbianism.* New York: Citadel.

Chafetz, J., Sampson, P., Beck, P., & West, J. (1974). A study of homosexual women. *Social Work, 19,* 714–723.

Cochran, S. D., & Mays, V. M. (1988). Disclosure of sexual preference to physicians by black lesbian and bisexual women. *Western Journal of Medicine, 149,* 616–619.

Council on Scientific Affairs. (1987). Aversion therapy. *Journal of the American Medical Association, 258,* 2562–2566.

Dardick, L., & Grady, K. E. (1980). Openness between gay persons and health professionals. *Annals of Internal Medicine, 93,* 115–119.

Deevey, S. (1990). Older lesbian women: An invisible minority. *Journal of Gerontological Nursing, 16*(5), 35–39.

Douglas, C. J., Kalman, C. M., & Kalman, T. P. (1985). Homophobia among physicians and nurses: An empirical study. *Hospital and Community Psychiatry, 36,* 1309–1311.

Doyle, T. L. (1967). Homosexuality and its treatment. *Nursing Outlook, 15*(8), 38–40.

Eliason, M. J., & Randall, C. E. (1991). Lesbian phobia in nursing students. *Western Journal of Nursing Research, 13,* 363–374.

Erlich, L. (1981). The pathogenic secret. In J. Chesebro (Ed.), *Gayspeak: Gay male and lesbian communication* (pp. 130–141). New York: Pilgrim Press.

Fisher, S., & Groce, S. B. (1985). Doctor–patient negotiation of cultural assumptions. *Sociology of Health and Illness, 7,* 342–374.

Garfinkle, E. M., & Morin, S. F. (1978). Psychologists' attitudes toward homosexual psychotherapy clients. *Journal of Social Issues, 34*(3), 101–112.

Glascock, E. L. (1981, November). *Access to the traditional health care system by nontraditional women: Perceptions of a cultural interaction.* Paper presented at the annual meeting of the American Public Health Association, Los Angeles.

Glascock, E. L. (1983, November). *Lesbians growing older: Self-identification, coming out, and health concerns.* Paper presented at the annual meeting of the American Public Health Association, Dallas.

Gonsiorek, J. C. (1988). Mental health issues of gay and lesbian adolescents. *Journal of Adolescent Health Care, 9*(2), 114–122.

Goodman, G., Lakey, G., Lashof, J., & Thorne, E. (1983). *No turning back: Lesbian and gay liberation for the '80s.* Philadelphia: New Society.

Hall, J. M., & Stevens, P. E. (1991). Rigor in feminist research. *Advances in Nursing Science, 13*(3), 16–29.

Harvey, S. M., Carr, C., & Bernheine, S. (1989). Lesbian mothers: Health care experiences. *Journal of Nurse-Midwifery, 34*(3), 115–119.

Hetrick, E. S., & Martin, A. D. (1987). Developmental issues and their resolution for gay and lesbian adolescents. *Journal of Homosexuality, 14*(1–2), 25–43.

Hume, B. J. (1983). *Perspectives on women's health: Disclosure decisions, needs, and experiences of lesbians.* Unpublished master's thesis, Yale University, New Haven, CT.

Hurst, M., & Zambrana, R. E. (1980). The health careers of urban women: A study in East Harlem. *Signs: Journal of Women in Culture and Society, 5*(3), S112–S126.

Jandt, F. E., & Darsey, J. (1981). Coming out as a communicative process. In J. Chesebro (Ed.), *Gayspeak: Gay male and lesbian communication* (pp. 12–27). New York: Pilgrim Press.

Johnson, S. R., Guenther, S. M., Laube, D. W., & Keettel, W. C. (1981). Factors influencing lesbian gynecological care: A preliminary study. *American Journal of Obstetrics and Gynecology, 140,* 20–28.

Jonas, S. (1974). Health, health care, and racism. *Hospitals, 48*(4), 72–75.

Jones, E. E., Farina, A., Hastorf, A. H., Markus, H., Miller, D. T., Scott, R. A., & French, R. (1984). *Social stigma: The psychology of marked relationships.* New York: W. H. Freeman.

Katz, J. N. (1976). *Gay American history: Lesbians and gay men in the U.S.A.* New York: Avon Books.

Katz, J. N. (1983). *Gay/lesbian almanac: A new documentary.* New York: Harper & Row.

La Fargue, J. P. (1972). Role of prejudice in rejection of health care. *Nursing Research, 21,*(1), 53–58.

Levy, T. (1978). *The lesbian: As perceived by mental health workers.* Unpublished doctoral dissertation, California School of Professional Psychology, San Diego.

Lewes, K. (1988). *The psychoanalytic theory of male homosexuality.* New York: Simon & Schuster.

Liljestrand, P., Gerling, E., & Saliba, P. A. (1978). The effects of social sex-role stereotypes and sexual orientation on psychotherapeutic outcomes. *Journal of Homosexuality, 3*(4), 361–372.

Liljestrand, P., Petersen, R. P., & Zellers, R. (1978). The relationship of assumption and knowledge of the homosexual orientation to the abridgement of civil liberties. *Journal of Homosexuality, 3*(3), 243–248.

Mathews, W. C., Booth, M. W., Turner, J. D., & Kessler, L. (1986). Physicians' attitudes toward homosexuality: Survey of a California county medical society. *Western Journal of Medicine, 144,* 106–110.

McGhee, R. D., & Owen, W. F. (1980). Medical aspects of homosexuality. *New England Journal of Medicine, 303,* 50–51.

Morin, S. F. (1977). Heterosexual bias in psychological research on lesbianism and male homosexuality. *American Psychologist, 32,* 629–637.

Moses, A. E. (1978). *Identity management in lesbian women.* New York: Praeger.

Nungesser, L. G. (1983). *Homosexual acts, actors, and identities.* New York: Praeger.

Olesker, E., & Walsh, L. V. (1984). Childbearing among lesbians: Are we meeting their needs? *Journal of Nurse-Midwifery, 29*(5), 322–329.

Owensby, N. M. (1940). Homosexuality and lesbianism treated with metrazol. *Journal of Nervous and Mental Disease, 92,* 65–66.

Paroski, P. A. (1987). Health care delivery and the concerns of gay and lesbian adolescents. *Journal of Adolescent Health Care, 8*(2), 188–192.

Randall, C. E. (1989). Lesbian phobia among BSN educators: A survey. *Journal of Nursing Education, 28,* 302–306.

Reagan, P. (1981). The interaction of health professionals and their lesbian clients. *Patient Counselling and Health Education, 3*(1), 21–25.

Robertiello, R. C. (1959). *Voyage from Lesbos: The psychoanalysis of a female homosexual.* New York: Citadel Press.

Romm, M. E. (1965). Sexuality and homosexuality in women. In J. Marmor (Ed.), *Sexual inversion: The multiple roots of homosexuality* (pp. 282–301). New York: Basic Books.

Roth, J. A. (1986). Some contingencies of the moral evaluation and control of clientele: The case of the hospital emergency service. In P. Conrad & R. Kern (Eds.), *The sociology of health and illness: Critical perspectives* (pp. 322–333). New York: St. Martin's Press.

Saghir, M. T., & Robins, E. (1973). *Male and female homosexuality: A comprehensive investigation.* Baltimore: Williams & Wilkins.

Saunders, J. M., Tupac, J. D., & MacCulloch, B. (1988). *A lesbian profile: A survey of 1000 lesbians.* West Hollywood, CA: Southern California Women for Understanding.

Schneider, B. E. (1982). Consciousness about sexual harassment among heterosexual and lesbian women workers. *Journal of Social Issues, 38*(4), 75–98.

Schneider, J. W., & Conrad, P. (1986). In the closet with illness: Epilepsy, stigma potential, and information control. In P. Conrad & R. Kern (Eds.), *The sociology of*

health and illness: Critical perspectives (pp. 110–121). New York: St. Martin's
Press.

Schwanberg, S. L. (1985). Changes in labeling homosexuality in health sciences literature: A preliminary investigation. *Journal of Homosexuality, 12*(1), 51–73.

Schwanberg, S. L. (1990). Attitudes towards homosexuality in American health care
literature 1983–1987. *Journal of Homosexuality, 19*(3), 117–136.

Seager, C. P. (1965, March 26). Aversion treatment in psychiatry. *Nursing Times*, pp.
423–424.

Shaw, C. T. (1971). A detailed examination of treatment procedures of whites and
blacks in hospitals. *Social Science and Medicine, 5*, 251–256.

Smith, E. M., Johnson, S. R., & Guenther, S. M. (1985). Health care attitudes and
experiences during gynecological care among lesbians and bisexuals. *American
Journal of Public Health, 75*, 1085–1087.

Socarides, C. W. (1968). *The overt homosexual*. New York: Grune & Stratton.

Stevens, P. E. (in press). Who gets care? Access to health care as an arena for nursing
action. *Scholarly Inquiry for Nursing Practice: An International Journal*.

Stevens, P. E., & Hall, J. M. (1988). Stigma, health beliefs, and experiences with health
care in lesbian women. *Image: Journal of Nursing Scholarship, 20*(2), 69–73.

Stevens, P. E., & Hall, J. M. (1990). Abusive health care interactions experienced by
lesbians: A case of institutional violence in the treatment of women. *Response: To
the Victimization of Women and Children, 13*(3), 23–27.

Stevens, P. E., & Hall, J. M. (1991). A critical historical analysis of the medical
construction of lesbianism. *International Journal of Health Services, 21*, 291–307.

Todd, A. D. (1989). *Intimate adversaries: Cultural conflict between doctors and women
patients*. Philadelphia: University of Pennsylvania Press.

Waitzkin, H. (1983). *The second sickness: Contradictions of capitalistic health care*.
New York: Free Press.

Waitzkin, H. B., & Waterman, B. (1974). *The exploitation of illness in capitalistic
society*. Indianapolis: Bobbs-Merrill.

Watters, A. T. (1986). Heterosexual bias in psychological research on lesbianism and
male homosexuality (1979–1983): Utilizing the bibliographic and taxonomic system
of Morin (1977). *Journal of Homosexuality, 13*(1), 35–58.

Wells, J. W., & Kline, W. B. (1987). Self-disclosure of homosexual orientation. *Journal
of Social Psychology, 127*(2), 191–197.

White, T. A. (1979). Attitudes of psychiatric nurses toward same sex orientations.
Nursing Research, 28(5), 276–281.

Wiesen-Cook, B. (1979). The historical denial of lesbianism. *Radical History Review,
20*, 60–65.

Wilbur, C. B. (1965). Clinical aspects of female homosexuality. In J. Marmor (Ed.),
Sexual inversion: The multiple roots of homosexuality (pp. 268–281). New York:
Basic Books.

Wolff, C. (1971). *Love between women*. New York: Harper & Row.

Young, E. W. (1988). Nurses' attitudes toward homosexuality: Analysis of change in
AIDS workshops. *Journal of Continuing Education in Nursing, 19*(1), 9–12.

Zeidenstein, L. (1990). Gynecological and childbearing needs of lesbians. *Journal of
Nurse-Midwifery, 35*(1), 10–18.

Zola, I. K. (1972). Medicine as an institution of social control. *Sociological Review, 20*,
487–504.

ECOLOGICAL TRANSITION: USING BRONFENBRENNER'S MODEL TO STUDY SEXUAL IDENTITY CHANGE

Judith Hollander, MSN, RN, CS
Veterans Affairs Medical Center, Fort Wayne, Indiana

Linda Haber, DNS, RN, CS
Veterans Affairs Medical Center, Marion, Indiana

Bronfenbrenner's (1979) ecological transition model provides a framework to study coming out in lesbians. The model takes into account activities such as sexual behavior, perceptions of the behavior, and social context in which behavior takes place. The importance of context makes this model useful in identifying possible connections between sexual identity alterations and larger social forces. Interventions based on this framework can reduce stress and promote health during coming out.

Sexual identity change or coming out is the process of adopting a lesbian or homosexual identity. It is developmental in nature, reflecting more or less permanent internal changes. The expression "coming out" suggests that the lesbian has always been inside, awaiting debut. Studies exploring lesbian identity formation reinforce the idea, describing what has been called the "gay trajectory" (Ponse, 1978), which includes a sense of being different and identification of the difference as a sexual-emotional attraction to other women (Elliott, 1985). However, in the 1970s, women who grew up with a subjective sense of being heterosexual, married, had children, and felt at home in the role of wife and mother also changed their sexual identity. The social context of the 1970s, which included rapid changes in values and community standards, may have contributed to the phenomenon of the previously het-

The authors thank Dr. I. Sue Bishop, Professor and Assistant Dean, Graduate Studies, College of Nursing, University of South Florida, for introducing them to Bronfenbrenner's model.

erosexual woman's coming out. In this article, we suggest a model that could be used to increase understanding of sexual identity change of both the traditional lesbian and the lesbian of the 1970s and to guide interventions and prevention strategies that facilitate a healthy movement to lesbian identity.

RELATED STUDIES

Although there has been little research on the transition to a lesbian or gay identity, several investigators have attempted to describe the process. The studies suggest that not only the homosexual behavior, but also the perception of the behavior and the context in which the behavior takes place are involved in the transition. The following discussion identifies significant studies that have increased our understanding of coming out.

The significance of the perception of sexual behavior in the coming-out process was initially identified by Dank (1971), who studied gay men. The study, replicated by Kus (1985), described a developmental process during which the individual undergoes a "cognitive shift" or change in how he views homosexual acts and his place within the homosexual life-style. Although a man may have been sexual with men, he would not identity himself as gay before the shift or change in perceptions. De Monteflores and Schultz (1978) and Cass (1979) included in their coming-out models for both lesbians and gays a necessary "cognitive transformation" comparable to Dank's shift. With this change, old actions take on new meanings.

But perceptions do not take place in a vacuum. Context participates in driving perception. Three examples of context's influencing perception of sexual behavior are sadomasochistic sexual activity, sex in prison, and homosexual acts within a heterosexual life-style.

Weinberg, Williams, and Moser (1984) studied sexual activity in a sadomasochistic subculture in California. Their data demonstrated that certain factors, including social content of the activity, must be present before the actor perceives it as sadomasochistic. In the absence of the appropriate environment, the activity might be perceived as sexual or violent but not sadomasochistic.

Sagarin (1976), studying homosexual activity of male prisoners, discovered that the "aggressor," the prisoner who initiated the act, did not perceive the act as homosexual, but as an assertion of masculinity. Female prisoners (Blumstein & Schwartz, 1976) interpreted homosexual activity not as lesbian, and at times not as sexual, but as a way to achieve nurturing. Again it was demonstrated that context contributed to the meaning of sexual activity.

Studies of men who engaged in both heterosexual and homosexual activities indicated that perception or evaluation of one's heterosexuality influences how homosexual activity is perceived (Hart, 1981). An active heterosexual context made it more difficult for an individual to adopt a homosexual identity (Paul, 1985; Troiden & Goode, 1980).

Thus, coming out is a cognitive process mediated by environmental or contextual factors. Dank (1971), investigating various social contexts in which change in sexual identity might occur, viewed contact and identification with the gay community as crucial to the cognitive shift. De Monteflores and Schultz (1978) conceptualized coming out "as a feedback loop regulating the relationship between the gay person and society" (p. 62), influenced by various personal and social factors. The ultimate result is change in sexual identity.

The literature exploring coming out suggests that homosexual/lesbian behavior, perception of that behavior, and the context in which the behavior takes place all influence the change. Any model used to examine coming out should attend to all three aspects. In his model of ecological transition, Bronfenbrenner (1979) viewed development as an alteration of an individual's position within his or her social environment. When developmental processes are explored, the model takes into account activities, perceptions, and social context; therefore, it contains the variables necessary to effectively examine coming out. The importance of context makes this model particularly useful in identifying possible connections between sexual identity alterations and social values changes such as those that existed in the 1970s.

THE MODEL

Our deliberation now proceeds to a presentation of ecological transition, a model that includes activities, perceptions, and social context and has the potential to identify both (a) components involved in the sexual identity change, including broad social factors, and (b) alterations that occur as a result of the new identity.

Sexual identity change can be conceptualized as an ecological transition in which the person's position within his or her social environment is altered as a result of changes in activities, roles, and interpersonal relationships (see Figure 1). Such changes are "both a consequence and an instigator of developmental processes requiring mutual accommodation between the organism and its surroundings" (Bronfenbrenner, 1979, p. 27). In other words, the changes in activities, roles, and relationships cause alterations that themselves may cause further shifts in activities, roles, and relationships. These changes are associated with disruption of settings and creation of new settings. From this perspec-

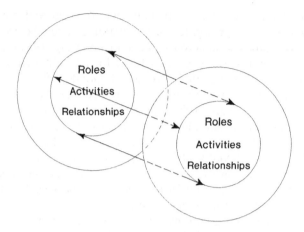

Figure 1. Sexual identity change is an ecological transition in which the person's position within his or her social environment is altered because of changes in activities, roles, and interpersonal relationships.

tive, change is viewed as a phenomenon that extends beyond the individual and his or her immediate environment.

Definition of Terms

In the ecological model, the environment is viewed as an arrangement of four nested subsystems in which the person develops by means of a process of interaction with the subsystems. Change, or ecological transition, can be instigated by pressure within any or all of the subsystems (see Figure 2). Setting and the four subsystems are defined as follows:

Setting—A setting is the context in which face-to-face interactions take place.

Microsystem—The most interior, or smallest, subsystem is the microsystem, defined as "a pattern of activities, roles, and interpersonal relations experienced by the developing person in a given setting" (Bronfenbrenner, 1979, p. 22).

Mesosystem—"A mesosystem comprises the interrelations among two or more settings in which the developing person actively participates" (Bronfenbrenner, 1979, p. 25). It is construed as the individual's social network.

Exosystem—The exosystem consists of settings in which the developing person is not an active participant "but in which events occur that affect, or are affected by, what happens in them" (Bronfenbrenner, 1979, p. 237). The exosystem comprises the larger community and includes such things as church doctrine and the legal system.

Macrosystem—The macrosystem refers to broad cultural issues and values that underlie the micro-, meso-, and exosystems.

Inherent in ecological transition is an emphasis not only on the objective properties of the environment but also on how the developing person perceives these properties. Perception of the environment rather than the objective environment is of primary importance because the meaning attributed by the participant steers his or her subsequent behavior (Bronfenbrenner, 1979).

Consequences of the Ecological Transition of Coming Out

The ecological transition of coming out involves multiple alterations in the individual's position in his or her social environment. These alterations reach beyond the immediate family or associates in the microsystem to impinge on the extended social network, or mesosystem. The effects of this transition may include (a) interruptions in relationships (e.g., parents, spouse, children, extended family, close friends, professional colleagues, and medical, legal, and religious representatives), (b) creation of new relationships (e.g., lesbian/gay friendships and development of relationships with sympathetic heterosexuals), (c) disruptions in settings (e.g., changing residence and socializing in different places), (d) development of new activities (e.g., changing church, job, and leisure-time pursuits), (e) the degree of internal conflict, and (f) the

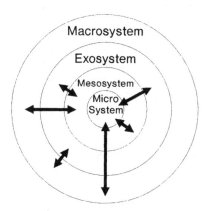

Figure 2. Pressure within any or all of the subsystems instigates ecological transition.

availability and change in availability of social support from the meso-system.

Usefulness of the Model

Extension of Knowledge

Ecological transition has the potential to extend knowledge about coming out. Its power lies in the explicit inclusion of the exosystem and macrosystem as sites of change. The exosystem and macrosystem of the 1970s are replete with study possibilities. The second wave of the women's movement, the anti-Vietnam movement, the civil rights movement, and developments in transportation and communication promoted and reflected change. These changes presented opportunities and pressures not previously encountered by women. Studies exploring these factors and their effects on women have the potential to expand our knowledge about sexual identity change. In addition, they can provide insight into the larger question of the relationship between forces originating in the exo- and macrosystems and individual development.

Framework for Interventions

Interventions based on the ecological transition of coming out could focus on any level of the environment, but can most easily address the micro- and mesosystems. Changes in roles, settings, and activities that occur at the microsystem level as a result of coming out may create a crisis. Interventions could be designed to facilitate effective coping, mitigate disruption in relationships, and promote development of new relationships. Educational programs aimed at what to expect as one comes out would help to alleviate the stress associated with confronting unknown situations.

The social network at the mesosystem level alters in response to changes in the microsystem. New individuals become part of the social network, while old friends leave. Members from the lesbian community may never be introduced to family and old friends. The social network will become more compartmentalized as fewer members of the social network know each other. As a result, the quantity and availability of social support will be modified. Interventions aimed at enhancing available social support will mitigate the stress associated with a changing life-style and promote healthy transitions (Hollander, 1989).

The exosystem consists of the larger community in which the lesbian and her social network reside. The legal system, as part of the exosystem, is a potential source of tension for the evolving lesbian. Legal issues that may arise for a woman undergoing a sexual identity change include divorce, issues of custody of minor children, co-parenting agreements, insurance, wills, and contracts. Educational interventions designed to smooth the way through legal conflicts will reduce stress.

In order for major changes in the exosystem to occur, the contents of the macrosystem, such as community standards and values, must be altered. The interactive nature of the exo- and macrosystems indicates that not only does change in values prompt change in laws, but also changes in laws facilitate value modification. For example, value changes in the 1950s and 1960s in the United States in regard to civil rights for blacks prompted legal upheaval that itself led to alterations in community standards. Research and education geared toward increasing public sensitivity to and awareness of lesbians may create a more sympathetic perspective about the whole issue of homosexuality. The arena would then be ripe for political activity aimed at creating a more equitable legal system for lesbians, which in turn would continue to influence community standards.

Mothers who come out will find shifts in all the systems. Interventions at the microsystem level could be aimed at mitigating stress associated with a changing family. Changes that occur as a result of divorce are applicable here: (a) single parenting, (b) integrating a new significant other into the family unit, (c) acknowledging their own and their children's grieving and loss, and (d) being estranged from family members (Bishop & Ingersoll, 1989). In addition to the usual tasks involved in the divorce transition, families that include lesbian mothers also need to cope with the mothers' and children's stigmatized identities. At the mesosystem level, assisting in the development of social networks that facilitate availability of social support for both children and mothers is critical.

In relation to mothering, the exosystem can be influenced by supporting a research agenda that explores the effects on children of being raised in an all-female household. Currently our knowledge is limited and influenced by unsubstantiated assumptions about the need for male role models within the home. Information gained from research has potential to alter the macrosystem and render lesbian parenting more acceptable.

Implications for Health Care Professionals

The essence of health care is the professional–client relationship. The quality of the relationship is determined largely by the professional's ability to be receptive to the client's needs. Negative attitudes interfere with the establishment of a quality helping relationship. Homosexuality in general and lesbianism in particular carry with them social stigma. Health care professionals, raised within this context, may have negative attitudes about lesbians, such as conceiving of them as sick or immoral. In Stevens and Hall's (1988) study, the majority of lesbians recounted negative responses from health care providers after disclosing their identity. Educating professionals about lesbians from an ecological perspective expands their base of understanding, allowing them to see all aspects of the life-style, including the process of coming out. The health care professionals will see that lesbians are multifaceted just like everyone else and not merely women who have sex with other women and will address their needs from this perspective (Smith, Heaton, & Seiver, 1990).

The ecological model provides the health care provider with a larger base from which to intervene, depending on interest and client need. For example, he or she can intervene in the mesosystem, advocating for ways to increase social support for the children. Viewing lesbianism and coming out at the exosystem level, professionals can establish a research agenda that increases knowledge about issues relevant to lesbians or can work for the development of policies and laws that facilitate a healthy lesbian life-style.

CONCLUSIONS

Because it includes both individual perception and the context of behavior as factors, the Bronfenbrenner (1979) model is useful in describing and explaining sexual identity change. We have presented recommendations for research and guidelines for interventions based on this framework. Future work with this model will help to increase both our understanding of sexual identity change and our ability to help women who are making this transition.

REFERENCES

Bishop, S., & Ingersoll, G. (1989). Effects of marital conflict and family structure on the self-concepts of pre- and early adolescents. *Journal of Youth and Adolescence, 18*(1), 25–38.

Blumstein, P., & Schwartz, P. (1976). Bisexuality in women. *Archives of Sexual Behavior, 5,* 171–181.

Bronfenbrenner, U. (1979). *The ecology of human development: Experiments by nature and design.* Cambridge, MA: Harvard University Press.

Cass, V. (1979). Homosexual identity formation: A theoretical model. *Journal of Homosexuality, 4,* 219–235.

Dank, B. (1971). Coming out in the gay world. *Psychiatry, 34,* 180–197.

De Monteflores, C., & Schultz, S. (1978). Coming out: Similarities and differences for lesbians and gay men. *Journal of Social Issues, 34,* 59–72.

Elliott, P. (1985). Theory and research on lesbian identity formation. *International Journal of Women's Studies, 8,* 64–71.

Hart, J. (1981). Theoretical explanations of practice. In J. Hart & D. Richardson (Eds.), *The theory and practice of homosexuality* (pp. 38–68). Boston: Routledge & Kegan Paul.

Hollander, J. (1989). Restructuring lesbian social networks: Evaluation of an intervention. *Journal of Gay and Lesbian Psychotherapy, 1*(2), 63–72.

Kus, R. (1985). Stages of coming out: An ethnographic approach. *Western Journal of Nursing Research, 7,* 177–198.

Paul, J. (1985). Bisexuality: Reassessing our paradigm of sexuality. *Journal of Homosexuality, 11,* 21–33.

Ponse, B. (1978). *Identities in the lesbian world: The social construction of the self.* Westport, CT: Greenwood.

Sagarin, E. (1976). Prison homosexuality and its effect on post-prison sexual behavior. *Psychiatry, 39,* 245–257.

Smith, M., Heaton, C., & Seiver, D. (1990, January). Health concerns of lesbians. *Physician Assistant,* pp. 81–94.

Stevens, P., & Hall, J. (1988). Stigma, health beliefs, and experiences with health care in lesbian women. *Image: Journal of Nursing Scholarship, 20*(2), 69–73.

Troiden, R., & Goode, E. (1980). Variables related to the acquisition of a gay identity. *Journal of Homosexuality, 5,* 382–392.

Weinberg, M., Williams, C., & Moser, C. (1984). The social constituents of sadomasochism. *Social Problems, 31,* 379–389.

Michele Eliason, PhD

College of Nursing, University of Iowa, Iowa City, Iowa

Carol Donelan, MA

Department of Comparative Literature, University of Massachusetts,
Amherst, Massachusetts

Carla Randall, MSN

Department of Nursing, Salish Kootenai Community College, Pablo, Montana

The American Psychological Association's Committee on Gay and Lesbian Concerns (Herek, 1987) expressed a need for research that focuses specifically on the concerns of lesbians. To this end, we attempted to identify stereotypes about lesbians, as noted in 278 female nursing students' responses to open-ended questions. Content analysis of the responses revealed a number of consistent themes or stereotypes. The most prevalent stereotypes included lesbians' seduction of heterosexual women, lesbian "boasting," and the "masculine aura" of lesbians. None of the participant variables (age, educational level, social class, and type of nursing education) were significantly related to particular stereotypes. The impact of stereotypes on the acceptance of lesbians within society is discussed.

In this article we describe negative attitudes expressed by nursing students about lesbians, show how these negative attitudes maintain stereotypes that oppress lesbians, and discuss how stereotypes may influence the quality of health care that lesbians receive.

In American society, lesbians have been described as "invisible women" (Guth, 1978), a reality that many lesbians themselves encourage and maintain out of necessity. Making oneself visible in a heterosexist society, in which the norm is heterosexual coupling and anything else

The authors thank Cheryl Cole, Ilene Alexander, and Nan Macy for their assistance with the development of this project.

is considered deviant, places a lesbian at risk for loss of family, children, job, and housing (Falk, 1989).

The heterosexist bias in society, which assumes that heterosexuality is the only "natural" alternative, promotes negative attitudes and stereotypes by emphasizing the ways lesbian behaviors, experiences, histories, and value systems differ from those of the dominant culture. The very existence of lesbians is construed as a threat to "traditional" values, which are founded on the subordination of women's needs, issues, and perspectives to those of men and on the denial of the potential bonds of love and friendship between women. A lesbian epistemology (ways of knowing the world) describes an alternative that focuses on the connections between women rather than viewing women in terms of men.

Academic research, imbued with the values of the dominant culture, contributes to lesbian invisibility in several ways. First, earlier studies on the topic of "homosexuality" often focused only on gay men or on "homosexuals" without addressing the specificity of lesbian existence (Anderson, 1981; Corbett, Troiden, & Dodder, 1977; Hudson & Ricketts, 1980; Lumby, 1976; Millham, San Miguel, & Kellogg, 1976; Smith, 1971). Much research has indicated that gay and lesbian lifestyles are sufficiently different to warrant separate study (Bell & Weinberg, 1978; Blumstein & Schwartz, 1983; Taylor, 1983).

Second, researchers who focused specifically on lesbians often examined questions of purported psychopathology rather than exploring the reasons why society does not accept lesbians (Caprio, 1954; Kaye et al., 1967). This blaming-the-victim approach has been noted in other research on marginalized groups as well (e.g., survivors of rape or incest) and contributes to the construction of negative stereotypes.

Finally, science is not objective, but is biased by the same heterosexist values as the nonscientific culture. Thus, any research concerning lesbian issues may be tainted with the same faulty assumptions that patriarchal society holds for women in general and lesbians in particular.

The Committee on Lesbian and Gay Concerns of the American Psychological Association (Herek, 1987) assigned high priority to "increasing commitment and APA attention to lesbian issues" (p. 3). Negative attitudes about lesbians prevalent in the dominant culture are one major concern. According to Pharr (1988), homophobia is one of the weapons of sexism, the system of institutional beliefs that keep women subordinate to men. Homophobia has been defined as an irrational fear of homosexuality. Because lesbians are perceived as a major threat to the patriarchy (they are not potential partners for men and do not follow traditional rules for women in this society), homophobia is encouraged by the system in order to keep lesbians invisible and powerless. Homophobia operates primarily through the maintenance of negative attitudes or stereotypes.

Stereotypes are based on the assumption that all members of certain social groups have inborn and unalterable characteristics, and thus the social construction of stereotypes is concealed. Stereotypes are, for the most part, demeaning and offensive and deny the recognition of individual differences among members of a group. Examples of stereotypes that act to condemn and censure lesbians include the "bull dyke," the "man hater," and the "predatory seductress" (Guth, 1978; Pharr, 1988). Some stereotypes are so pervasive in the media and popular culture that they are assumed to be true, not only by people outside the stereotyped group, but by those within the group as well (referred to as "internalized homophobia" when lesbians believe negative stereotypes about themselves). Because stereotypes are generally based on partial truths, or are true for small subsets of a marginalized group, they are easily maintained and generalized. For example, lesbians who choose to adopt certain behaviors or appearances that signify "lesbian" according to prevalent (and for the most part, negative) stereotypes make themselves visible to the dominant culture and reinforce the stereotype. These visible lesbians are often subject to homophobic reactions from their families, friends, or co-workers. Such reactions may be built on feelings of anxiety, disgust, aversion, anger, discomfort, and fear. Others choose to remain invisible to avoid experiencing the homophobic reactions of others.

Homophobia in various helping professions, including psychology, medicine, social work, and nursing, has detrimental effects for lesbians seeking care from such professionals (Davison & Wilson, 1973; Humphreys, 1983; Levitt & Klassen, 1974; MacDonald & Games, 1974; White, 1979). Lesbians often reported that health care providers were judgmental, nonsupportive, and negative toward them if they revealed their sexual orientation (Chafetz, Sampson, Beck, & West, 1974; Smith, Johnson, & Guenther, 1985). Stevens and Hall (1988) found that although lesbians wanted to disclose their lesbian identity to health care providers, they usually did not for fear of retaliation and poor quality of care. Brossart (1979) wrote that female nurses were particularly threatened by lesbians because "they'd be afraid of what others might suspect if they appeared to be accepting of her" (p. 49). Randall (1987) found that nurse educators did not include discussions of lesbian health care issues in either the classroom or the clinical setting.

The silence about lesbian issues in health care training, whether due to lack of knowledge or to homophobia, perpetuates the invisibility of lesbians and may contribute to poorer quality of care by neglecting to inform health care providers of the unique needs of lesbians.

We had two aims in the present study. First, we wanted to identify the common stereotypes about lesbians held by one segment of the health care community—female nursing students. Identifying stereotypes is an important first step in planning interventions to reduce or deconstruct the stereotypes. We wish to emphasize our underlying assumption that stereotypes are socially constructed (e.g., Kitzinger, 1987). Close examination of stereotypes might provide insight into the faulty beliefs that underlie the stereotype and provide means of altering these beliefs via education or social action.

The second aim of the study was to explore potential underlying factors that may contribute to homophobia, such as age, education, and social class status of study participants. A goal of nursing education is to recruit women and men who are nurturing and accepting of diversity, suggesting that nursing students as a whole might be more accepting of lesbians. On the other hand, nursing continues to be defined as a traditional female career and attracts a large number of women (primarily white and middle class) who have conservative views of women's roles. Samples of nursing students often contain a large percentage of women with high self-endorsed "feminine" characteristics, such as caringness, yieldingness, sympathy, sensitivity, and compassion (Eliason & Randall, 1991). Previous research has suggested that highly "feminine" women are more threatened and less accepting of sex role difference than "androgynous" or "masculine" women (Bem, 1987; Black & Stevenson, 1984). Research has also suggested that women are less tolerant of lesbians and men are less tolerant of gay men (Kite, 1984; Whitley, 1987). Thus, "feminine" women may be at high risk for negative attitudes toward lesbians.

Other potential underlying factors of homophobia include age and educational level. Herek (1984) found greater age and education to be related to greater acceptance of gays and lesbians, whereas Randall (1987) found no such relationship. However, the two studies had quite different samples and methods of gauging acceptance.

METHOD

Subjects

Two hundred ninety-four nursing students participated in the study. The majority fell into the age group of 19–22; however, they represented a wide age range (19–48) and all levels of nursing education, from first-year prenursing majors to students with nearly completed graduate degrees. The participants were drawn from three different types of nursing education programs: a community college, a small private college, and a major university nursing program. The sample included 16 male and 278 female students. The sample was 96% white, and 82% identified themselves as middle or upper class. Only 2% identified themselves as lesbians. Male nursing students' questionnaires were excluded from the analysis because of the small number.

Procedure

After students were invited to participate, and written consent forms were signed, each participant was asked to complete a questionnaire that included demographic information, the Bem Sex Role Inventory (Bem, 1974), a series of questions on political issues, and an experimental manipulation (ratings of photographs of women labeled as lesbians). The findings and complete procedures are described elsewhere (Eliason & Randall, 1991). Of present interest are the responses to three open-ended questions:

1. How would you know if a co-worker was a lesbian?
2. How would you feel about working with a woman you knew to be a lesbian?
3. Are lesbians a threat to society?

Open-ended questions were selected because much of the earlier research on homophobia used behavioral checklists or true–false statements about "homosexuals" to identify stereotypes. This method does not allow participants to articulate attitudes in their own words. Also, the previous emphasis on "homosexuals" with questions that assumed gay men and lesbians were the same may have obscured any unique attitudes toward either lesbians or gay men. These open-ended questions also provided a specific context in which to respond—working with a lesbian in a health care setting.

In this sample, 68% responded to at least one of the three questions. Nonresponding may have been related to a number of factors, such as no opinion on the topic, uneasiness about the questions, lack of time, or other factors. The results are based on the sample of 189 participants who responded to at least one of the open-ended questions. These participants did not differ from the nonresponders on age, social class, educational level, or Bem scores.

A content analysis of the responses to the open-ended questions was conducted to determine common themes or patterns that might represent stereotypes. Two of the investigators independently rated the questions for themes to establish reliability. Agreement on major themes was greater than 95%.

RESULTS

The findings are presented in two sections. First, the themes identified by the content analysis are described, and examples of responses are provided for validation. The percentages reported are based on the 189 participants who responded to one or more of the questions. In the second section, factors that may have been related to development of these stereotypes are discussed. These factors include participant's type of nursing education, age, and social class identification.

Recurrent Themes in the Group as a Whole

Several major themes emerged from the survey results. The majority of these themes attributed a range of negative behaviors to lesbians. Very few neutral or positive themes were identified.

The most prevalent theme was that lesbians aim to seduce heterosexual women. A large segment of the sample (38%) suggested that heterosexual women should be wary of sexual advances by lesbians. Respondents suggested "keeping a distance" from all lesbians to "protect" themselves from those "overly friendly" lesbians who will "make eyes at you" or "put the moves on you." Related to the notion of lesbian aggressiveness toward other women was the idea that lesbians preach their life-style to others and do not respect the choices heterosexual women make in regard to sexual relationships. Twenty-nine percent of the sample suggested that lesbian "proselytizing" was something to contend with and that lesbians would be "better off" if they would "stop trying to push their beliefs" on heterosexual women. References to partners or activities in the lesbian community was equated with "boasting" about "exploits." In a work setting, lesbians who discussed their social lives with co-workers or indicated the nature of their social or sexual relationships outside the workplace were considered "too pushy," "preachy," or "insensitive." "I would hope that this type of woman would respect me and others and not talk about her life-style freely," wrote one participant. Two participants feared that "normal human beings" can "contract" lesbianism "like a contagious disease" through the various forms of lesbian proselytizing. "They are sick," wrote one respondent. "They are not normal human beings. They try to turn young, normal people into lesbians with their gay marches."

Many respondents expressed feelings of "unease," "anxiety," "discomfort," and "distrust" around lesbians who indicated through various means that they were lesbian. Three percent of the sample suggested that lesbians "flaunt" their life-style in "gross" or "inappropriate public displays" of affection.

In response to the question "How would you know if a co-worker was a lesbian?", 26% of the respondents stated that lesbians were identifiable only through self-disclosure. However, 31% suggested that lesbians may be picked out of a crowd based on their "aura of masculinity." Features that supposedly set lesbians apart from heterosexual women include "masculine" or "out of style" dress, "jeans, heavy boots, flannel shirts, leather coats," "wallets with chains," "manly, athletic, short-cropped hair," "hairy underarms," and "lack of make-up." One respondent wrote that lesbians are "ugly women who can't get dates with men" while another identified a lesbian as "a woman who clings to other women and puts men down all the time."

The issue of acquired immune deficiency syndrome (AIDS) is of particular interest in this survey of future health care providers. In spite of increasing AIDS education in nursing school curricula, 13% of the respondents identified lesbians as responsible for the spread of AIDS. Respondents also noted that lesbian acts produce or encourage the spread of "infectuous [sic], sexually transmitted diseases" other than AIDS.

Fourteen percent of the survey participants expressed the view that lesbianism is biologically unnatural. According to one respondent, lesbianism "destroys the traditional ideal of heterosexuality" and is therefore "against human nature." Others objected to homosexual relationships because of the "inability of gays and lesbians to reproduce."

Closely allied with those who objected to lesbianism as "biologically unnatural" were the 13% who objected to lesbianism on moral, ethical, or religious grounds. More often than not, these respondents based their objections on passages from the Bible. One participant wrote, "I believe in the Bible, and the Bible says homosexuality is wrong. Besides, why did God make two sexes? If people were to be homosexual, God would have made one sex." Another respondent suggested that lesbianism "destroys society's sense of morality and virtue" and "makes the world a worse place in which to live." Objections to lesbianism on religious grounds were often based on the "pleasure without purpose" principle. "What's the point of lesbian love, except for pleasure?" queried one respondent. "God made men and women to love each other and multiply for the sake of continuing our society and culture." Lesbian relationships were also viewed as a "threat to the propulsion [sic] of the Christian family."

Some respondents (11%) wrote that lesbians provide negative role models for children and were concerned about the negative influence lesbians might have on children. A small minority (3%) objected to lesbian relationships on the basis of an "incomplete family unit."

Although the notion of "rampant lesbian sexuality" was a common belief among the respondents, only 3 participants directly accused lesbians of child molestation. Other infrequent themes in the data were that lesbians are nonconformists (4%); that if too many women became lesbians, there would not be enough women for men to marry (3%); and that lesbians hate men (3%).

Factors Related to Lesbian Stereotypes

A number of demographic and personality variables were examined in relation to negative attitudes. Type of nursing education program (major university vs. small private college vs. community college) seemed to have no effect. Because virtually identical patterns of response were noted in the three samples, they were combined for further analyses.

Some researchers have found that negative attitudes decrease as age increases, supposedly as a result of increased experience and exposure to societal diversity. However, in this sample, very few stereotypes changed significantly with age. Fewer older female nursing students denounced lesbianism on the basis of religion or moral judgments, and older students were somewhat less likely to identify lesbians as seducers of heterosexual women. Other themes remained fairly stable across age groups. However, there were relatively few participants in the older age range (only 38 participants were over 40 years of age, whereas 122 participants were ages 19–22).

DISCUSSION

Several common themes or patterns representing current stereotypes about lesbians were identified in this sample of female nursing students. The most prevalent of these themes and their possible social origins are discussed below.

"Lesbians Seduce Heterosexual Women"

The most common theme was fear of seduction, perhaps reflecting a stereotype of lesbian sexual assertiveness. Sexual assertiveness is typically considered a "masculine" gender trait, not a characteristic appropriate for women to display in a patriarchal society. Because lesbian sex is independent of men and of reproductive functions, it is construed as "other" than traditional female sexuality. In this heterosexist society, sexuality is a dichotomous variable: There is male sexuality and there is female sexuality. If a lesbian is not perceived as fitting within female sexuality as defined by the culture, then, according to the sexual dichotomy, she must be construed as representing male sexuality. Young women may (realistically) fear seduction by men and may generalize that fear to lesbians. This sample may also be expressing a developmental fear of sexuality. More than 50% of the sample was under the age of 25, a time of exploration of one's own sexuality and need to conform to influential others. Any behavior that deviates from the narrow "norm" may be viewed as threatening.

"Lesbians Want To Be Men"

More than 30% of the sample suggested that lesbians could be readily identified by their masculine style of dress, hairstyle, or mannerisms. Because no respondent mentioned any "feminine" characteristics of lesbians, this sample appeared to believe that lesbians as a group are more likely to look and act like men. This equating of lesbians with masculine traits may be due to the higher visibility of lesbians who choose to wear more androgynous or stereotypically male attire, whether for political or comfort reasons. Some lesbians also behave in ways more commonly allocated to men in our society (e.g., independence, participation in athletics, and nontraditional occupational choices). This subset of more visible lesbians may interpret their own behavior as a challenge to the status quo or as a self-affirming choice, whereas the heterosexual population appears to interpret this behavior as proof that lesbians want to be men. Lesbians who are more feminine in their appearance and behavior are less visible and thus do not contribute to the stereotype.

"Lesbians Are Too Blatant"

Many respondents strongly object to lesbians' talking about their life-styles. Some participants did suggest that "it's okay as long as they keep it to themselves," but many complained that lesbians try to preach their life-styles and do not respect the choices of others. Respondents did not want lesbians to mention their private lives in the workplace or reveal any hint of their lesbianism in public. If a lesbian talked about her life-style in the same manner as heterosexual co-workers, she was accused of being "too pushy." This homophobic attitude contributes to the large number of lesbians who remain closeted for fear of society's rejection. Such a theme may not represent a stereotype per se, but provides an example of "tolerance" for lesbian life-styles without acceptance. Blumenfeld and Raymond (1988) argued that mere tolerance actually promotes lesbian invisibility and allows for discriminatory practices to occur. They suggested that tolerance masks a basic underlying fear or hatred in individuals who cognitively support civil rights, but emotionally cannot accept lesbian sexuality. Tolerance is extended to children or immature individuals, thus often representing a condescending attitude.

"Lesbians Are a Bad Influence on Children"

The stereotype that lesbians are a bad influence on children was reported by 11% of the sample. However, the myth of child molestation was noted on only 3 respondents' questionnaires. Perhaps this stereotype is slowly disappearing, dispelled by statistics that show that heterosexual males are by far the most common perpetrators of sexual abuse of children (Brownmiller, 1975). However, the high endorsement of a sexual aggressiveness stereotype might suggest otherwise. The young age of the respondents (primarily single and childless women) might be related to the lower frequency of this stereotype in this particular sample.

"Lesbians Spread Sexually Transmitted Diseases"

Previous research has identified a "disease" stereotype regarding "homosexual" activity. However, a new myth of the 1980s and 1990s appears to be that lesbians are a common source of AIDS as well as other sexually transmitted diseases. More than 13% of the sample made explicit mention of AIDS in the open-ended questions. Even more participants (28%) endorsed agreement with the statement that "Lesbians are a high risk group for AIDS" on another section of the questionnaire (Eliason & Randall, 1991). Randall (1987) found that 18% of nurse educators in her sample also thought that lesbians were a common source of AIDS, suggesting that nursing students are not being provided with accurate information in the classroom. Many authors have suggested that the heterosexual society tends to consider gay men and lesbians as a homogeneous group. However, considerable differences in lifestyles have been noted, and lesbians are still less likely to engage in unsafe sexual practices than most other groups, putting them at lower risk for sexually transmitted diseases than gay men or heterosexual couples (Loulan & Burton-Nelson, 1987). There is ample evidence that lesbians have lower rates of gonorrhea, syphilis, and chlamydia than heterosexual women (Johnson, Guenther, Laube, & Keettel, 1981; Masters & Johnson, 1979; Robertson & Schacter, 1981). Much of the current theory and practice suggests that AIDS education needs to focus on high-risk behaviors, not groups of people. As this goal is accomplished, perceptions of risk groups may change.

Factors Related to Stereotypes

Age of respondents was largely uninformative. On the whole, the same stereotypes were found in all age groups. The only themes that tended to decline in frequency in the older group were the denouncement of lesbianism on the basis of religious beliefs and the lesbian seduction stereotype. The differences across age groups were relatively small.

Our previous research (Eliason & Randall, 1991) and that of others (e.g., Herek, 1984) suggested that one of the few predictive factors in positive attitudes toward gay men or lesbians was familiarity. In the current sample, nursing students who reported knowing a lesbian had more accepting attitudes. However, the majority (70%) indicated that they did not know any lesbians, attesting to the invisibility of many lesbians. This invisibility presents a real dilemma for attempts to reduce negative stereotypes. Familiarity with lesbians (particularly those in the "invisible" category) helps to dispel stereotypes, yet the fear of loss of job, family, and friendships that accompanies negative stereotypes helps to maintain lesbian invisibility, keeping the pool of visible lesbians small.

In addition to the preceding concerns, the current political climate, a very vocal and wealthy fundamentalist Christian minority, and a Supreme Court that is systematically restricting rights of marginalized groups by undermining or overruling civil rights legislation combine to maintain negative stereotypes about lesbians. The conservative climate may negate any gains made by greater visibility and inclusion of lesbians and gays in political campaigns, legislative agendas, textbooks, and the media in general.

CONCLUSION

Because of limitations in the sample (only female nursing students) and the method (open-ended questions for which 32% of the sample did not provide answers), the stereotypes identified in this study need to be reidentified in a larger and more heterogenous sample. However, it is likely that these negative attitudes are pervasive in this society with its heterosexism and historical emphasis on traditional sex role behavior.

Nursing students are bound to the nursing code of ethics, which states, "The nurse provides services with respect for human dignity and the uniqueness of the client unrestricted by considerations of social or economic status, personal attributes, or the nature of health problems." The type of negative attitudes identified in this study are clearly contradictory to this code of nursing ethics. The contradiction needs to be challenged in the classroom and in practice. In nursing, as well as in other helping professions, it appears that deviations from accepted sex role behaviors may be thought exempt from codes of ethics or considerations of human rights. Education aimed at dispelling stereotypes and providing accurate information about lesbian cultures is desperately needed in the helping professions.

Finally, acknowledgment of lesbian stereotypes as social constructions used by a patriarchal society to keep women in general and lesbians in particular invisible and powerless may help to direct future intervention-based research onto a more productive path. Psychological research and educational practices need to take into account feminist readings of the social, economic, and political climates in which these stereotypes flourish.

REFERENCES

Anderson, C. L. (1981). The effect of a workshop on attitudes of female nursing students toward male homosexuality. *Journal of Homosexuality, 7,* 57–69.

Bell, A. P., & Weinberg, M. S. (1978). *Homosexualities.* New York: Simon & Schuster.

Bem, S. L. (1974). The measurement of psychological androgyny. *Journal of Consulting and Clinical Psychology, 42,* 155–162.

Bem, S. L. (1987). Probing the promise of androgyny. In M. R. Walsh (Ed.), *The psychology of women* (pp. 206–225). New Haven, CT: Yale University Press.

Black, K. N., & Stevenson, M. R. (1984). The relationship of self-reported sex-role characteristics and attitudes toward homosexuality. *Journal of Homosexuality, 9,* 83–93.

Blumenfeld, W. J., & Raymond, D. (1988). *Looking at gay and lesbian life.* New York: Philosophical Library.

Blumstein, P., & Schwartz, P. (1983). *American couples: Monies, work, sex.* New York: William Morrow.

Brossart, G. (1979). The gay patient: What you should be doing. *RN, 42*(4), 50–52.

Brownmiller, S. (1975). *Against our will.* New York: Simon & Schuster.

Caprio, F. (1954). *Female homosexuality.* New York: Citadel.

Chafetz, J., Sampson, P., Beck, P., & West, J. (1974). A study of homosexual women. *Social Work, 19,* 714–723.

Corbett, S. L., Troiden, R. R., & Dodder, R. A. (1977). Tolerance as a correlate of experience with stigma: The case of the homosexual. *Journal of Homosexuality, 3,* 3–13.

Davison, G. G., & Wilson, T. G. (1973). Attitudes of behavior therapists toward homosexuality. *Behavior Therapy, 4,* 686–696.

Eliason, M. J., & Randall, C. E. (1991). Lesbian phobia in nursing students. *Western Journal of Nursing Research, 13,* 363–374.

Falk, F. J. (1989). Lesbian mothers: Psychosocial assumptions in family law. *American Psychologist, 44,* 941–947.

Guth, J. T. (1978). Invisible women: Lesbians in America. *Journal of Sex Education and Therapy, 4*(1), 3-6.

Herek, G. M. (1984). Beyond "homophobia": A social psychological perspective on attitudes towards lesbians and gay men. *Journal of Homosexuality, 10,* 1-21.

Herek, G. M. (1987). *Committee on Lesbian and Gay Concerns Report to the American Psychological Association.* Washington, DC: American Psychological Association.

Hudson, W. W., & Ricketts, W. A. (1980). A strategy for the measurement of homophobia. *Journal of Homosexuality, 5,* 357-372.

Humphreys, G. E. (1983). Inclusion of content on homosexuality in the social work curriculum. *Journal of Education in Social Work, 19,* 55-60.

Johnson, S. R., Guenther, S. M., Laube, D. W., & Keettel, W. C. (1981). Factors influencing lesbian gynecologic care: A preliminary study. *American Journal of Obstetrics and Gynecology, 140,* 20-28.

Kaye, H., Berl, S., Clare, J., Eleston, M., Gershwin, B., Gershwin, P., Kogan, L., Torda, C. & Wilbur, C. (1967). Homosexuality in women. *Archives of General Psychiatry, 17,* 626-634.

Kite, M. E. (1984). Sex differences in attitudes toward homosexuals: A meta-analytic review. *Journal of Homosexuality, 10,* 69-81.

Kitzinger, C. (1987). *The social construction of lesbianism.* London: Sage.

Levitt, E. E., & Klassen, A. D., Jr. (1974). Public attitudes toward homosexuality: Part of the 1970 national survey by the Institute for Sex Research. *Journal of Homosexuality, 1,* 29-43.

Loulan, J., & Burton-Nelson, M. (1987). *Lesbian passion: Loving ourselves and each other.* San Francisco, CA: Spinsters/Aunt Lute.

Lumby, M. E. (1976). Homophobia: The quest for a valid scale. *Journal of Homosexuality, 2,* 39-47.

MacDonald, A., & Games, R. (1974). Some characteristics of those who hold positive and negative attitudes toward homosexuals. *Journal of Homosexuality, 1,* 9-27.

Masters, W. & Johnson, V. (1979). *Homosexuality in perspective.* Boston: Little, Brown.

Millham, J., San Miguel, C. L., & Kellogg, R. (1976). A factor-analytic conceptualization of attitudes toward male and female homosexuals. *Journal of Homosexuality, 2,* 3-10.

Pharr, S. (1988). *Homophobia: A weapon of sexism.* Inverness, CA: Chardon.

Randall, C. E. (1987). Lesbian-phobia among BSN educators: A survey. *Cassandra: Radical Nurses' Journal, 6,* 23-26.

Robertson, P. & Schachter, J. (1981). Failure to identify venereal disease in a lesbian population. *Sexually Transmitted Diseases, 8,* 75-79.

Smith, E., Johnson, S., & Guenther, S. (1985). Health care attitudes and experiences during gynecologic care among lesbians and bisexuals. *American Journal of Public Health, 75,* 1085-1087.

Smith, K. T. (1971). Homophobia: A tentative personality profile. *Psychological Reports, 29,* 1091-1094.

Stevens, P. E., & Hall, J. M. (1988). Stigma, health beliefs, and experiences with health care in lesbian women. *Image: Journal of Nursing Scholarship, 20*(2), 69-73.

Taylor, A. (1983). Conceptions of masculinity and femininity as a basis for stereotypes of male and female homosexuals. In M. W. Ross (Ed.), *Homosexuality and social sex roles* (pp. 37–53). New York: Haworth.

White, T. A. (1979). Attitudes of psychiatric nurses toward same-sex orientations. *Nursing Research, 28*(5), 276–281.

Whitley, R. E. (1987). The relationship of sex-role orientation to heterosexuals' attitudes toward homosexuals. *Sex Roles, 17,* 103–113.

REASONS AMERICAN LESBIANS FAIL
TO SEEK TRADITIONAL HEALTH CARE

Susan E. Trippet, RN, DSN, and Joyce Bain, RN, EdD
School of Nursing, University of Southern Mississippi, Hattiesburg, Mississippi

What reasons do lesbians have for not seeking health care? From three women's cultural events in 1990, a convenience sample was formed of 503 women (78% of whom were lesbians) who volunteered to complete a pretested qualitative and quantitative instrument. The reasons given for not seeking health care from traditional sources were that (a) low-cost, natural, or alternative care is not provided; (b) holistic care is not provided; (c) little preventive care and education are provided; (d) communication and respect are lacking; and (e) there are few women-managed clinics.

Culturally sensitive health care is needed for several different populations and particularly for hidden populations. Lesbians may be considered a hidden population because one cannot tell by looking at or physically examining a woman what her sexual orientation is. She may or may not reveal her orientation in response to a direct question. As a result, lesbians have not been identified in most studies of women's health care. Studies involving homosexuals sometimes include lesbian women, as though same-sex-oriented men and women could be compared equally. Lesbians perceive themselves differently from the way opposite-sex-oriented women or same-sex-oriented men perceive themselves (Stevens & Hall, 1988). Unlike other groups of women, lesbians are isolated from society through society's homophobia and general stigmatization. Lesbians tend to hide their differences for fear of recrimination and retaliation from society.

The conceptual framework for the present study was feminist theory as outlined by Fee (1975), Gilligan (1982), and Miller (1976). According to feminist theory, women deserve access to the same choices available to men, and the access should not be mediated by sex, age, race, or socioeconomic barriers. Health care is but one of the arenas where ac-

---

This study was funded in part by Sigma Theta Tau, Gamma Lambda chapter.

cess and interactional dynamics exist and are managed within a patriarchal system. Access to health care in the United States is controlled by the American Medical Association, insurance companies, legislatures (medical and nursing practice legislation), and individual communities' political systems. All of these systems are dominated by men. Because women interact from a relational stance (Gilligan, 1982; Miller, 1976), they are acutely aware of the interactional dynamics of communication. A major concern of lesbians is the lack of communicated awareness and sensitivity of health care providers. Reported negative health care experiences have contributed to lesbians' choosing Eastern and ancient health practices rather than Western practices.

REVIEW OF THE LITERATURE

In a review of 22 years of literature on lesbians' health concerns, the paucity of research was evident. Only four studies were published in refereed journals; a fifth study was published privately.

Johnson, Guenther, Laube, and Keettel (1981) conducted a preliminary study with 117 lesbians to identify health care use, gynecological and obstetrical problems, and attitudes toward physicians. The lesbians were young (under 35 years old) and well educated. The researchers found that a number of the women sought alternative sources for health care and speculated whether some of the women sought any health care at all. Johnson et al. could only make educated guesses as to why lesbians did not seek care.

In the follow-up study (Johnson, Smith, & Guenther, 1987; Smith, Johnson, & Guenther, 1985), the researchers queried 1,921 lesbians and 424 bisexuals during a women's cultural event in 1980. The majority of women were young, white, middle class, college educated, and from urban areas. One of the findings was that use of alternative health care correlated with the women's personal beliefs that disclosure of sexual orientation would negatively affect the quality of health care received from physicians.

Reagan (1981) recruited 38 lesbians for the purpose of discovering the relationships and attitudes of lesbians to health care providers. Her participants were young, well-educated women who used private physicians. Reagan suggested that sexual orientation issues contributed to lesbians' delay in seeking health care. The women predicted that health care providers would react negatively to a client if they knew she was a lesbian, and that the lesbians feared the providers' responses.

In a more recent study, Stevens and Hall (1988) used a qualitative method with 25 lesbians to explore the relationship between health and lesbianism and lesbians' interactional experiences with health care providers. The lesbians were young, white, college educated, and employed. Health was characterized as being holistic, and lesbians valued and nurtured their sense of independence and self-reliance as being important to wellness. The majority of experiences with health care providers were negative and occurred within various settings. Several comments by women were presented that suggested possible reasons why lesbians did not seek health care. There was no mention of whether the lesbians rejected or delayed seeking health care.

Bradford and Ryan (1989) conducted a study with 1,925 lesbians from all 50 states. The researchers wanted to discover the health and health care needs of lesbians throughout the United States. Typically, the majority of lesbians were young, college educated, middle class, and employed. Reasons for failing to seek health care were explored. The two major reasons cited were the lesbians' participation in self-care (as a result of negative experiences with health care providers) and the lack of financial resources.

Our review of the literature guided us in our attempt to expand and update the data on lesbian women's health concerns. Our purpose in conducting the 1990 study was to identify and explore the physical and mental health concerns of lesbians and bisexual women. During the pilot testing of the instrument in 1989, we discovered that lesbians did not consistently seek health care when they needed it (Trippet & Bain, 1990). This information led us to explore why lesbians failed to seek health care.

METHOD

The pretested instrument, Physical and Mental Health Concerns of Lesbians, was based on the research by Johnson et al. (1981, 1987) and Smith et al. (1985) and included additional categories of family and social issues, mental health concerns, and legal aspects (Trippet & Bain, 1990). The instrument contained both qualitative and quantitative items for content analysis and descriptive statistics.

Collecting data from an invisible population could pose a problem in that there are only a few places where lesbians may be found in large numbers. One of these places is a women's cultural event. We selected three women's cultural events from which data could be collected—two in the southeastern United States and one in the midwest—all of which occurred during the spring of 1990. Permission to collect data was secured from the University of Southern Mississippi and the sponsors of each event.

The procedure for data collection included setting up a table with chairs in a convenient location of traffic flow during the event. Signs announced the research, and we orally described the research to potential volunteers.

Frequency, percentage, and chi-square analyses were performed on the quantitative data. The three samples were tested for homogeneity and were found to be homogeneous. Qualitative data on the open-ended questions were initially coded into categories, and frequencies of responses were identified. The inductive process was used to determine higher level categories and their respective frequencies.

RESULTS

Sample

A convenience sample of 503 women volunteered to complete the instrument. They were white (92.8%, n = 467), under the age of 40 (68.8%, n = 346), and college educated (75.8%, n = 381) and represented 38 states. Seventy-five percent (n = 377) of the women earned more than $15,000 annually. These demographic characteristics reflect the same profile as that in other research with lesbians (Bradford & Ryan, 1989; Johnson et al., 1981, 1987; Reagan, 1981; Smith et al., 1985; Stevens & Hall, 1988; Trippet & Bain, 1990), essentially those lesbians who are out or halfway out of the closet.

Although many of the women had a health care provider that they saw annually or biannually, 24.7% (n = 124) failed to seek health care. Of those who did seek health care, 77.1% (n = 388) chose a private physician, 17.5% (n = 88) a woman's center, 13.1% (n = 66) homeopathic care, and 12.7% (n = 64) a nurse practitioner. Other health care providers were rated more positively than physicians, especially male physicians.

Health care providers are not meeting the needs of lesbian women. The reasons lesbians gave for not seeking health care from traditional sources were that (a) low-cost, natural, or alternative care is not provided; (b) holistic care is not provided; (c) little preventive care and education are provided; (d) communication and respect are lacking; and (e) few women-managed clinics are available.

Low-Cost Natural Alternatives

Reasons why lesbians did not seek health care were inferred from how lesbians viewed their health care experiences and what they would like to see changed in physical health care. The women were clear about what they wanted in health care. Being unsatisfied with the current Western medical approaches of medication and surgery, they sought alternative health practices that are less invasive and more in tune with the human body and nature. Specific examples of what these lesbians wanted include

> More alternatives—acupuncturist, chiropractic, whole body approach, nutrition, and more insurance coverage for each. More lesbian gynecologists.

> More women, more natural and home remedies, more herbs; use food as natural medicine, not just entertainment.

Health care and health insurance are expensive for women. Alternative approaches such as homeopathic and naturopathic practitioners, acupuncturists, and chiropractors are less expensive but are not reimbursed by most insurance companies. Only a few states have statutes that allow the reimbursement of nurse practitioners.

Holistic Health Care

The present lesbians had obviously spent time learning about themselves and trying to integrate their same-sex sexual orientation into society's opposite-sex sexual orientation. Perhaps their quest for integration led them into literature, individual reflection, and group discussions concerning health. Or perhaps they were just tracing the history of our foremothers in believing that the body, mind, and spirit work in concert with the environment. At any rate, they arrived at the need for holistic health care through some intellectual process. Their comments reflect the need for holism in health care. They want

> more care centered on the whole individual, . . . encourage people to heal themselves. I hate patriarchal medical views on womyn—the narcotics prescribed—the needless, disfiguring surgeries done.

> Utilization of holistic health care—the mind–body–environment connection. Use herbology, . . . techi/shiaism [shiatsuism—acupressure]/yoga, macrobiotics, etc.

> I would like to have one particular primary health care provider (preferably a lesbian nurse practitioner or nurse-midwife) who would be reimbursed by my insurance company for routine preventive care and only be referred to specialists as needed.

> Less organ removal, more herbal, more of a balance between Eastern and Western philosophies.

> Health care should be more mutual. Massage, herbal care, [and] chiropractors should be accepted health care.

> *Prevention* vs. crisis interventions.

Preventive Health Care and Education

The last comment leads into the third reason these lesbians did not seek traditional health care. A common complaint was that too little time is spent on preventive health care and preventive education. Also, the lesbians voiced the need for providers to give more emphasis to women's issues and medical problems. The following comments highlight the need for preventive education and care:

> All doctors need to get back to nutritional diets and get the patient involved.

> More information about potential problems of [the] uterus; encourage lesbians to get regular gynecologic care (I didn't because birth control was not applicable), i.e., items of concern to me were infrequent periods with heavy flow. Over years, various family doctors told me—nothing to worry about. When I saw a gynecologist, he identified those as risk factors for cancer. If I'd known that earlier, I would have gone to the gynecologist earlier. As it is, they got it all surgically, but I can't help wondering if earlier treatment could have alleviated or avoided it.

Poor Communication and Lack of Respect

The complaint of increased need for preventive care occurred concomitantly with providers' poor communication and lack of respect. Frustration and anger concerning providers' lack of personal regard and attendance to personal need are evident in the following comments:

> Practitioners need to learn to *listen* to clients—*share lots* of information, listen for unasked questions and fears (especially related to anger) and do not assume heterosexuality! Also, [they] need to know or care about lesbian health concerns.

> More time spent with me—willingness to explain in lay terms what's happening during an exam and what the results [are].

> Patients "allowed" to make their own decisions regarding treatment. Not asking irrelevant questions on medical questionnaires—i.e., whether or not I have been pregnant *is* a valid question, whether or not I am married is *not* relevant to my health—only behavior.

> Listen to womyn! We know ourselves and our bodies!

These women felt the lack of respect from traditional health providers, and some of them turned to alternative health providers for respect, complete information, preventive care, and collaborative decision making regarding their health care.

Women-Managed Clinics

The lesbians also wanted women- or nurse-practitioner-managed clinics available to them for health care. More female health providers was the most frequent request. Although some lesbians would prefer a lesbian provider, the gender of the provider was more important than the sexual orientation. They felt more comfortable with female practitioners, as do many women regardless of sexual orientation. Some of their comments were specific:

> More women's centers or nurse practitioners available in rural areas.

> Natural, holistic health care centers run by women. More accessible women's clinics that actually have women doctors.

Summary

Underlying all five reasons for lesbians' failing to seek traditional health care was the fear of discrimination or the actual experience of discrimination from health providers toward lesbians as women and as lesbians. Although the five reasons appear to be reasons all women would have in seeking health care, the natural–alternative practices seem to belong to a small segment of the adult female population. Lesbians and a growing number of heterosexual women are developing a different relationship with their environment and with people. They view the pollution of the environment on a global and a personal level. They want as few chemicals around or near them as possible and announce that need by permitting no aerosols, no perfumes, no drugs, no alcohol, and no smoking in a specified area during women's cultural events. These women consider perfume and scented cosmetics as potential stimulation for allergies and asthma attacks.

CONCLUSIONS

The nursing profession has a role to play in meeting the health needs of culturally sensitive populations. Within women-managed clinics, nurse practitioners can provide alternative health practices such as herbal and natural therapies, creative visualization, biofeedback, and massage. In many cases, these strategies can be tried before medications are given or invasive techniques are attempted.

Nurses are the usual source for preventive health education. They are the ones who teach breast self-examination and the need for annual Pap smears. The teaching role can be expanded to meet the needs of lesbians by a holistic approach involving the body, mind, and spirit. Nurses and physicians can take the time to listen carefully to the cues clients give them; exploration of those cues may lead them to a more accurate diagnosis and treatment of the problem. Involvement of the client in any decision making is essential. Health care in its most effective form is an interdependent, mutual process.

Clinics and provider offices need a file of education materials on all health subjects that arise. The materials must be written in lay language, even though these women are highly motivated to use medical libraries where they are available. Most important, health care providers need to remember that heterosexuality is but one form of sexual expression. If the suggested strategies are not implemented, it seems clear that lesbians will continue to avoid traditional health care facilities or perhaps care of any kind.

The present findings can be generalized only to lesbians in the United States. Even that may be an overgeneralization because this study and all others conducted with lesbians sample only those women who are accessible, those who are out or halfway out of the closet, and who are white, middle class, and well educated. Numerous strategies have been explored to modify the methodological problem, without success. As long as homophobia exists or is perceived, methodological problems will continue to exist.

REFERENCES

Bradford, J., & Ryan, C. (1989). *The national lesbian health care survey: Final report.* Washington, DC: National Lesbian and Gay Health Foundation.

Fee, E. (1975). Women and health care: A comparison of theories. *International Journal of Health Services, 5,* 397–415.

Gilligan, C. (1982). *In a different voice: Psychological theory and women's development.* Cambridge, MA: Harvard University Press.

Johnson, S. R., Guenther, S. M., Laube, D. W., & Keettel, W. C. (1981). Factors influencing lesbian gynecologic care: A preliminary study. *American Journal of Obstetrics and Gynecology, 140,* 20–25.

Johnson, S. R., Smith, E. M., & Guenther, S. M. (1987). Comparison of gynecologic health care problems between lesbians and bisexual women: A survey of 2,345 women. *Journal of Reproductive Medicine, 32,* 805–811.

Miller, J. B. (1976). *Toward a new psychology of women.* Boston: Beacon.

Reagan, P. (1981). Lesbian women and their relationship to health professionals. *Patient Counselling and Health Education, 3,* 21–25.

Smith, E. M., Johnson, S. R., & Guenther, S. M. (1985). Health care attitudes and experiences during gynecologic care among lesbians and bisexuals. *American Journal of Public Health, 75,* 1085–1087.

Stevens, P., & Hall, J. (1988). Stigma, health beliefs, and experiences with health care in lesbian women. *Image: Journal of Nursing Scholarship, 20,* 69–73.

Trippet, S. E., & Bain, J. (1990). Preliminary study of lesbian health concerns. *Health Values: Health Behavior, Education, & Promotion, 14*(6), 30–36.

LESBIANS AS AN INVISIBLE MINORITY IN THE HEALTH SERVICES ARENA

M. Morag Robertson, MS, RNC, OGNP
Penquis Family Planning, Bangor, Maine

Ten self-identified lesbians were interviewed about their health care experiences. Analysis of the data from a grounded theory approach revealed four issues: health care providers' assumption of heterosexuality, reactions to coming out, lesbians' expectations of health care, and health-care-seeking behavior. It is the invisibility of lesbians in society that lends to the continued negative experiences lesbians relate. As health care professionals, we must assess our present practices and seek ways to improve the quality of care we offer to lesbians. Some recommendations for improving care to the lesbian community are made.

The delivery and accessibility of health care services are sociopolitical issues today. The elderly, the poor, and minorities are struggling to maintain adequate health care. Lesbians are one of the minorities, although an invisible minority.

The traditional health care system has based its care and treatment of women on assumptions of heterosexuality (Bernhard & Dan, 1986; Dardick & Grady, 1980; Johnson, Guenther, Laube, & Keettel, 1981; Stevens & Hall, 1988). The assumption is that all women are heterosexual, unless stated otherwise. As Good (1976) noted, many physicians believe they have never treated a lesbian. In order to provide appropriate gynecological diagnosis and treatment, accurate information pertaining to a woman's sexual activity and orientation is important. Unfortunately, some researchers have found that lesbians put off seeking medical care or risk potential misdiagnosis because of fear of potential negative reactions from the provider (Dardick & Grady, 1980; Reagan, 1981). In addition, because of the lack of knowledge about lesbian health needs (O'Donnell, 1978), providers are left to rely on information pertaining to heterosexual women.

The health care concerns of lesbians differ from those of heterosexual women. My purpose in conducting this study was to add to the present knowledge base regarding lesbian health care; describe whether assumptions of heterosexuality are made by the provider and whether this assumption adversely affects the lesbian health care experience; suggest ways to provide nonheterosexist care; and describe the health care experiences of lesbians.

LITERATURE REVIEW

There is a paucity of research on the health care experiences of lesbians. Before the removal of homosexuality in the second edition of the *Diagnostic and Statistical Manual of Mental Disorders* (American Psychiatric Association, 1973) in 1973, research focused on the "causes" of and "treatment" for homosexuality. Within the last 10 years, researchers have looked at the roles of the gynecologist and the lesbian client (Good, 1976; Johnson et al., 1981; Johnson & Palermo, 1984). There are signs that nurses and other health professionals are beginning to conduct research on the health needs of lesbians (Hepburn & Gutierrez, 1988; Stevens & Hall, 1988), but the studies are few.

Good (1976) surveyed 110 gynecologists in Dade County, Florida. Surprisingly, he found that more than 50% had not knowingly treated a lesbian. This would seem unlikely, considering that the estimate of female homosexuality by Kinsey (1953) is approximately 5%. More recent figures place the lesbian population at a minimum of 10% (Goodman, Lakey, Lashof, & Thorne, 1983). Good did presume lesbians may prefer a female provider. However, Good surveyed 6 of the 7 female gynecologists and found again that 50% stated that they had never provided care to a lesbian. Furthermore, Good asked the physicians how they knew whether a patient was a lesbian. Out of the 72 who stated they had treated at least one lesbian, 25 claimed to be able to tell by using clinical observation and judgment. One has to wonder what special skills these gynecologists had that allowed for such observations without asking the woman directly. Only 9 physicians had asked about the woman's sexual orientation, but 38 said that the patient had provided the information.

The assumption of heterosexuality on the part of the health care provider has recently been documented (Dardick & Grady, 1980; Johnson & Palermo, 1984; Reagan, 1981; Stevens & Hall, 1988). One area in which this assumption occurs is birth control. Typically, the respondent was asked if she was sexually active and, if so, what form of birth control she used. Some respondents also reported that the medical history assumed heterosexuality. The language of the questions that applied to marital status and sexual activity were noted by some of the respondents as areas of concern (Dardick & Grady, 1980; Johnson & Palermo, 1984).

In addition, Stevens and Hall (1988) noted that 72% of their respondents had experienced a negative reaction when they disclosed their sexual preference. Examples reflected shock, embarrassment, and fear on the part of the provider. Reagan (1981) identified an even more harmful outcome. Twenty-four percent of the lesbians in this study had at one time delayed care because of concerns regarding negative responses to their sexual preference. Smith, Johnson, and Guenther (1985) categorized the negative responses. They noted that the respondents described various reactions by the health care provider, and only 58% who had disclosed their sexual orientation responded to this question. The negative responses from health professionals included cool (12%); embarrassed (30%); inappropriate (25%), described as voyeuristic or suggesting a referral to a mental health professional; and overt rejection (22%), for example, "He got up, left the room, and had a nurse finish the questioning." Both female and male providers were found to respond equally in a negative manner. The findings by Stevens and Hall (1988) lend support to this earlier study. These negative reactions must be acknowledged in order for all health care providers to overcome their own prejudices and biases.

Johnson and Guenther (1987) discussed the importance of coming out to a health care provider. "Coming out" means identifying oneself as gay or lesbian. Lesbians and gay men have stated that coming out to a provider is essential, as documented in studies by Dardick and Grady (1980), Johnson et al. (1981), and Smith et al. (1985). The samples in the studies were not random, and thus this finding lacks generalizability. This does not diminish the significance of the finding, however.

What sources of health care do lesbians use? Johnson and Palermo (1984) found that 35% of their respondents sought nontraditonal or alternative care. However, alternative care was not defined, and no mention was made about the sources of care for the other 65%. On the other hand, specific sources of health care were identified by Johnson et al. (1981) and Smith et al. (1985): 38% and 55% used gynecologists or family practitioners, 17% and 10% student health services, and 45% and 34% alternative settings, respectively. The alternative sites included women's health clinics and offices of nurse practitioners and chiropractors. It would seem that physicians and nurses provide care for lesbians, but the providers are not aware of the sexual preference of some of these women.

Johnson and Palermo (1984), Johnson et al. (1981), and Smith et al. (1985) identified some of the barriers lesbians face when seeking health care. They must endure assumptions of heterosexuality, negative reactions, inadequate care, disregard for partners, and issues surrounding confidentiality. The dilemma therefore is, Does one identify oneself as a lesbian in order to receive adequate care, or risk potential adverse consequences?

METHOD

My aim in conducting this study was to describe lesbians' health care experiences from their perspective. The grounded theory approach developed by Glaser and Strauss (1967) was used. In this approach, the incoming data are coded and compared using a constant comparative method. This allows for the emergence of categories of data to illustrate specific concepts. With continued data gathering, along with literature review for support, properties of the categories are identified. It is from these properties that a hypothesis is developed (Stern & Pyles, 1986).

To conduct the study, I developed a semistructured interview containing open-ended questions. The questions were pilot tested on a small sample $(N = 5)$, refined, and then evaluated for content validity by the participants. The final questions were as follows:

1. Can you tell me about your experience as a lesbian in seeking health care?
2. Did your identification have any effect on the care, and if so can you describe this?
3. Do you have a preference in regard to a health care provider?
4. Have you had any experiences with a partner? If so, can you tell me about them?
5. Have you ever not sought health care because of your sexual orientation? If so, can you describe why?

A nonrandom sample of 10 self-identified lesbians was recruited by word of mouth by providers working in a health care setting known to provide care to the lesbian and gay community (7) and also by the researcher (3). All the participants were white, had at least a high school education, were ages 26–40, and were working full- or part-time. Most had health insurance. An obvious bias with this self-selected group is the lack of representation of women of color and the fact that the majority of respondents were identified in a gay-sensitive health center.

Seven respondents were interviewed in the health care clinic, and 3 were interviewed in the their homes. The interviews lasted approximately 1 hr and were audiotaped and later transcribed. After I completed transcription, I erased the audiotape.

The incoming data were processed, coded, and categorized as each interview was completed. As the analysis of the data continued, four themes emerged. A property of two themes was the assumption of the health professional that a woman is heterosexual unless she states otherwise. This assumption led to a core variable, the invisibility of lesbians within society, which allows for the perpetuation of negative experiences.

RESULTS

Assumption of Heterosexuality

The assumption of heterosexuality was a dominant theme throughout the interviews. Not surprisingly, the two most common areas in regard to this were contraceptive needs and sexual activity. Two respondents expressed their confusion in attempting to answer these questions.

> I might have said yes [to being sexually active] and they said do you need birth control. I said no. Maybe they were a little confused. I could have also said no, thinking well it's not real sex, you know, to them.

> I think it just confused them. I remember they just didn't believe me when I said I was sexually active but I wasn't using birth control, I didn't need any birth control, and I didn't need any birth control information from them, so that was probably confusing for them.

In addition, one respondent expressed her concern regarding the difficulty in answering these questions: "You hope they don't ask, you know, like what's going on in your sex life, because you're going to have to answer or lie."

Two participants spoke about the health history questionnaire:

> When I filled out a health history form it said, "Sexually active, yes; type of birth control, none." When I went into her office she said you're sexually active and not using birth control, and I said, "Yes. I live with a woman."

> In answering the questions, are you sexually active and do you use birth control, I just write down I'm a lesbian and that they are very heterosexist questions and that they need to change their questionnaire.

The designers of questionnaires continue to assume that all women are heterosexual and thus require contraception.

Coming Out

Self-identification as a lesbian encompassed the providers' reaction to this information and how the respondent felt. It should be noted that those women who came out to providers were more comfortable with their sexual identity.

> I don't have a problem with my sexuality so I don't really have a problem telling people that I have a partner.

> I don't know if it is because it is a woman, you know, that I was more comfortable in coming out or if it was because I knew her, or that I'm more comfortable with myself.

The majority of reactions from providers when some identified themselves as lesbian were "fine." However, two respondents commented on the nonverbal cues: "She was a little taken aback" and "They'd kind of look away." Furthermore, two women detailed negative and inappropriate reactions.

> When I told her that I was a lesbian she said do you want an AIDS test.

> I identified myself lesbian to one and the reaction was very bad, really bad. Saying "that is not natural, that's against God's law, maybe you should think a little bit harder about what you're doing." And he tried to give me a moral lecture on the evils and sins of lesbianism and how wrong I was and was young and there was time to repent.

Once these women came out to the provider, feelings of being "exposed," "embarrassed," and "less anonymous" and of a "void" in the experience were common. Two respondents felt that their examinations were "rushed": "I feel like she was in a hurry to get rid of me as a patient"; "They blow it off and do a quicker exam." One woman's experience with an obstetrician left her feeling her medical complaint was psychologically based: "I really left her feeling something was wrong with me mentally rather than physically." Finally, one respondent spoke of her experience with a partner.

> So I went in with her and I was completely discounted . . . she couldn't understand why I was there. She asked me about three times why was I there. It was harder for me to help her than probably it would have been if I had been a man sitting there with her and had a legitimate relationship to this person.

Expectations

All of the respondents had expectations in regard to their health care experiences. A female provider was the preference of all respondents. The provider did not need to be a lesbian, but must be comfortable and sensitive to lesbian health issues. The respondents wanted a provider who "listens" and is "knowledgeable," "competent," "understanding," and "sensitive to lesbian issues." One participant summed it up by saying,

> Health care! A health care provider who's comfortable with herself and comfortable with us. The same thing anybody else wants. I just want someone who is competent, understanding, and caring.

Health-Care-Seeking Behavior

This final category included the frequency with which care was sought and the reasons routine care was not a part of the health care experience.

> I think one . . . of the obstacles for me in terms of health care is like getting myself there and paying for it. Money is always a factor and time because usually, you know, I have to take off work or something to come in or when an appointment is available.

> You put it off because nobody is harassing you to do it. I don't think it's a conscious decision not to.

> I don't feel like I need to go. I don't feel like I need to go on a yearly basis. I don't feel like I'm at risk for cervical cancer.

None of the respondents received any routine health care, and some felt yearly examinations were not necessary.

CONCLUSIONS

Equal access to health care is a right. Today in the United States many go without care because of lack of insurance; lack of financial resources; and, in some instances, discrimination. This study identified some of the barriers lesbians face. It is important to note that the providers for most of the respondents were physicians. Nevertheless, all health care providers should consider their present practice and seek ways to respond to the lesbian community.

Health professionals must recognize that lesbians have concerns that differ from those of heterosexual women and continue to speak to those needs with further research. Health care providers first need to assess the present knowledge base in regard to lesbian health issues. An integral element is acknowledging the presence of prejudicial attitudes, myths, and stereotypes (Jones, 1988; Pogoncheff, 1979) and how they influence the lesbian experience. In speaking with lesbians about their life-styles and experiences, caregivers will gain insight and knowledge

72   M. M. Robertson

that will help direct quality care (Edelman, 1986; Gillow & Davis, 1987).

The findings of this study correspond with the findings of previous researchers (Johnson & Guenther, 1987; Johnson et al., 1981; Smith et al., 1985; Stevens & Hall, 1988). The assumption of heterosexuality by the health care provider poses a problem for the lesbian seeking care. Does she disclose her sexual orientation and risk the consequences of a negative reaction or no reaction, or does she lie about her sexual orientation out of fear? This study served to identify the invisibility of lesbians and how this invisibility adversely affects their health care experiences.

A more deleterious outcome is to delay care or seek no care at all out of fear of health providers' reactions. Do lesbians also fail to seek routine care for financial reasons, or, as one respondent expressed, because of believed low risk? As health care providers, we have a responsibility to educate all women about the importance of preventive health measures, which include routine screening examinations.

An additional finding of this study is that all the respondents preferred female providers. Because the majority of nurses are women, we are in a unique position to improve the lesbian health care experience. To accomplish this, we must work toward educating our peers and other providers about lesbian issues. Further, if we create an atmosphere that is open, supportive, nonjudgmental, and nonheterosexist, lesbians will have access to care that is free from some of the obvious barriers that persist today. Women's health concerns, including those of lesbians, must continue to be addressed and valued as important areas of research.

REFERENCES

American Psychiatric Association. (1973). *Diagnostic and statistical manual of mental disorders* (2nd ed.). Washington, DC: Author.

Bernhard, L., & Dan, A. (1986). Redefining sexuality from women's own experiences. *Nursing Clinics of North America, 21*, 123–136.

Dardick, L., & Grady, K. (1980). Openness between gay persons and health professionals. *Annals of Internal Medicine, 93*, 115–119.

Edelman, D. (1986). University health services sponsoring lesbian health workshops: Implications and accessibility. *Journal of American College Health, 35*(1), 44–45.

Gillow, K., & Davis, L. (1987). Lesbian stress and coping methods. *Journal of Psychosocial Nursing, 25*(9), 28–32.

Glaser, B., & Strauss, A. (1967). *The discovery of grounded theory: Strategies for qualitative research.* Hawthorne, NY: Aldine de Gruyter.

Good, R. (1976). The gynecologist and the lesbian. *Clinical Obstetrics and Gynecology, 19*, 473–481.

Goodman, G., Lakey, G., Lashof, J., & Thorne, E. (1983). *No Turning Back: Lesbian and gay liberation for the '80s.* Philadelphia: New Society.

Hepburn, C., & Gutierrez, B. (1988). *Alive and well: A lesbian health guide.* Freedom, CA: Crossing Press.

Johnson, S., & Guenther, S. (1987). The role of "coming out" by the lesbian in the physician–patient relationship. *Women and Therapy, 6*(1–2), 231–238.

Johnson, S., Guenther, S., Laube, D., & Keettel, W. (1981). Factors influencing lesbian gynecological care: A preliminary study. *American Journal of Obstetrics and Gynecology, 140,* 20–28.

Johnson, S., & Palermo, J. (1984). Gynecological care for the lesbian. *Clinical Obstetrics and Gynecology, 27,* 724–730.

Jones, R. (1988). With respect to lesbians. *Nursing Times, 84*(20), 48–49.

Kinsey, A. (1953). *Sexual behavior in the human female.* Philadelphia: W. B. Saunders.

O'Donnell, M. (1978). *Lesbian health matters.* Santa Cruz, CA: Santa Cruz Women's Health Center.

Pogoncheff, E. (1979, April). The gay patient. *RN,* pp. 46–52.

Reagan, P. (1981). The interaction of health professionals and their lesbian clients. *Patient Counselling and Health Education, 3,* 21–25.

Smith, E., Johnson, S., & Guenther, S. (1985). Healthcare attitudes and experiences during gynecological care among lesbians and bisexuals. *American Journal of Public Health, 75,* 1085–1087.

Stern, P. N., & Pyles, S. H. (1986). Using grounded theory methodology to study women's culturally based decisions about health. In P. N. Stern (Ed.), *Women, health, and culture* (pp. 1–24). Washington, DC: Hemisphere.

Stevens, P., & Hall, J. (1988). Stigma, health beliefs, and experiences with health care in lesbian women. *Image: Journal of Nursing Scholarship, 20*(2), 69–73.

HEALTH LIFE-STYLES OF LESBIAN
AND HETEROSEXUAL WOMEN

Julie A. Buenting, RNC, CNM, DNS
Brockport, New York

In this exploratory descriptive study, lesbian and heterosexual wom-
en's health life-style activities and health histories were investigated. Distribution of 200 written questionnaires by nonprobability
snowball sampling obtained a sample of 79 heterosexual and lesbian
women. The sample was predominantly white, middle class, and
college educated. Responses to questions about participation in
mental health counseling, birth control use, and pregnancy history
showed significant differences between the groups. Likert scale
questions were used to identify degree of participation in various
health life-style activities. Alternative diet, use of meditation/
relaxation techniques, and recreational drug use had significantly
higher means in the lesbian group. Fulfilling family obligations,
regular Pap testing, and use of prescription drugs were significantly
higher among the heterosexual group. This study represents the
author's initial exploration of lesbian health life-styles and describes
similarities and differences in the health life-styles of lesbian and
heterosexual women.

The feminist women's health movement has drawn attention to numerous problems and inadequacies in the health care system. One such
problem is that lesbian women have often been invisible and ignored by
health care providers, educators, and researchers. The limited professional literature about lesbian women's health has been fragmented in its
approach to health issues and has often reflected heterosexist attitudes
and deviance-based views of lesbianism. Previous medical and nursing
authors have demonstrated a conceptualization of lesbianism rooted in
illness or deviance models by emphasizing research concerning etiology

The author thanks Peggy L. Chinn, RN, PhD, FAAN; Charlene Eldridge Wheeler, RN,
MS; and Clarice Lechner-Hyman, RN, EdD for their guidance in this research.

(Dritz, 1980), substance abuse (Diamond & Wilsnack, 1978; Lewis, Saghir, & Robins, 1982), and sexually transmitted diseases (Johnson & Palermo, 1984; Robertson & Schachter, 1981). Other studies have examined women's health care use patterns (Good, 1976; Johnson, Guenther, Laube, & Keettel, 1981) or their relationships with health care providers (Smith, Johnson, & Guenther, 1985; Stevens & Hall, 1988).

Recently health care providers and researchers have recognized the need for greater understanding of health issues important to lesbian women. Several authors have investigated lesbian women's childbearing plans (Johnson, Smith, & Guenther, 1987) and lesbian women's experiences within the health care system when choosing childbearing (Harvey, Carr, & Bernheime, 1989; Olesker & Walsh, 1984; Wismont & Reame, 1989). Despite these preliminary efforts to address lesbian health issues, many gaps remain in our knowledge of lesbian women's experiences of health. In this exploratory descriptive study, I intended to increase our understanding of lesbian women's health by comparing the health life-style activities and health histories of lesbian and heterosexual women.

METHOD

Participants

A nonprobability sample of adult women was recruited from the Rochester and Buffalo metropolitan and suburban areas in western New York. Snowball sampling was used, and 200 written questionnaires were distributed through women's bookstores, community groups, and gay and lesbian organizations. Participants completed the questionnaires and returned them by mail. Participation could be entirely anonymous, but those respondents who revealed their identity were assured of confidentiality.

The sample obtained consisted of 79 women, with the majority indicating white race, middle socioeconomic class, college-level education, and current employment. On the basis of self-reported sexual partner preference, 34% ($n = 27$) of the 79 were assigned to the lesbian group, and 66% ($n = 52$) were assigned to the heterosexual group. The age range for the total sample was 20–66 years, with a mean age of 35.9. The lesbian group was younger, ranging from 21 to 43 years, with a mean age of 28.7, while the heterosexual group ranged in age from 20 to 66 years, with a mean age of 39.7. This difference between the two groups was statistically significant by t test, $t(77) = 5.31$, $p < .001$. No significant differences were found between the groups for other demographic characteristics.

Materials

A written questionnaire was developed specifically for this study. The questionnaire instrument used fixed-alternative questions to gather demographic information, health history data, and self-reports of social interaction patterns and sexual partner preference. Health life-style activity data were obtained using questions that asked respondents to indicate the degree to which various health-related and illness-screening activities were a part of their life-style on a 4-point Likert scale, from *not a part of my life-style* (1) to *a very central part of my life-style* (4). Additional health history questions investigated participation in mental health counseling, birth control use, pregnancy history, and description of general health status.

The questionnaire instrument was assessed for face, content, and construct validity by a panel of nurse educators before pilot testing. After pilot testing was completed, minor revisions in question wording, format, and instructions were made to increase clarity and ease of completion.

RESULTS

Health life-style activity items for the Likert scale were selected with consideration for incorporating a holistic conceptualization of health activities and including interpersonal and spiritual activities as meaningful health activities. The Likert scale items were analyzed using *t* testing. The Likert scale format was used for the following 14 items of health life-style activity: regular exercise, alternative diet, abstinence from alcohol, drinking alcohol, fulfilling family obligations, use of recreational drugs, use of prescribed medications, use of meditation/relaxation techniques, religious/spiritual activities, monthly breast self-examination, community service, regular Pap tests, smoking cigarettes, and social activities.

In this sample, *t* testing demonstrated statistically significant differences between the lesbian and heterosexual groups for the health lifestyle activities alternative diet, regular Pap tests, use of meditation/relaxation techniques, use of recreational drugs, use of prescription drugs, and fulfilling family obligations. The lesbian group showed significantly higher mean scores on alternative diet, meditation/relaxation techniques, and use of recreational drugs. The heterosexual group demonstrated higher mean scores on regular Pap tests, use of prescribed medications, and fulfilling family obligations.

Eight of the health life-style activity Likert items did not show a significant difference between the lesbian and heterosexual groups.

These items were regular exercise, smoking cigarettes, community service, social activities, monthly breast self-examination, religious/spiritual activities, abstinence from alcohol, and drinking alcohol. Table 1 presents group means and t statistics for the health life-style Likert scale items that were significantly different between the two groups.

Questionnaire respondents were asked to indicate whether they had ever participated in mental health counseling or therapy. Nearly three fourths (74%) of the lesbian group reported having attended some form of therapy or counseling, and two thirds of the heterosexual group had done so. Chi-square analysis with Yates correction for continuity revealed this difference to be statistically significant, χ^2 (1, $N = 78$) = 8.447, $p < .01$.

Additional health history information was collected concerning birth control use. More than 80% of the heterosexual women (42 of 50) reported past or current birth control use, compared with 47% (12 of 26) of the lesbian group. This difference was also statistically significant according to chi-square analysis with Yates correction, χ^2 (1, $N = 76$) = 10.129, $p < .01$. In both groups the most frequently used method was the oral contraceptive, followed by the diaphragm.

Differences were found in pregnancy history between the two groups. Of the heterosexual participants, 13 (26.5%) reported one pregnancy, 10 (20.4%) reported two pregnancies, 9 (18.3%) reported three pregnancies, and 5 (10.1%) reported four or more pregnancies. Only 2 lesbian participants reported pregnancies: One woman had had a pregnancy that

Table 1. Health Life Style Activity Statistics

Life-style activity	Lesbian		Heterosexual		
	M	SD	M	SD	$t(76)$
Regular Pap tests	2.15	0.82	3.12	0.86	4.91****[a]
Meditation	2.37	1.08	1.71	0.90	−2.73***
Use of prescribed medications	1.56	1.00	2.12	1.03	2.26*
Use of recreational drugs	1.56	0.69	1.18	0.52	−2.48**
Fulfilling family obligations	2.92	0.74	3.48	0.77	3.07***
Alternative diet	2.33	1.14	1.78	1.04	−2.09*[b]

[a]$df = 77$, not 76.
[b]$df = 75$, not 76.
*$p < .05$.
**$p < .02$.
***$p < .01$.
****$p < .001$.

was terminated, and another lesbian woman reported two full-term pregnancies and births. The percentage of women planning pregnancy was identical in each group. Four women in the heterosexual group (7.6%) and two women in the lesbian group (7.6%) were planning to seek pregnancy in the near future.

A final health history question asked respondents to indicate their general health status. The majority of respondents in both groups characterized their general health status as excellent or good, and no statistically significant difference was found between the groups using chi-square analysis, χ^2 (3, $N = 77$) = 0.952, $p = ns$.

DISCUSSION

This study represented an initial exploration of the health life-styles of lesbian and heterosexual women. Although health care providers might assume initially that the health life-style activities of lesbian and heterosexual women would be quite different, in this study I found both similarities and differences between the two groups.

The significant difference between the groups in Pap test frequency is consistent with Smith et al.'s (1985) finding that lesbian women are less likely to seek routine gynecological care. This may reflect a perception among lesbian women that regular Pap tests are unnecessary unless one is heterosexually active, or it may be an age-related difference because of recent debate over recommended intervals for Pap testing. Alternately, less frequent participation in Pap smears and routine gynecological examination may indicate that the lesbian women have had or expect to have negative experiences in their interactions with gynecological care providers.

Significant differences were found between the lesbian and heterosexual groups in the use of prescribed and recreational drugs. These differences may be somewhat age-related, however. The mean scores of both groups for use of prescribed and recreational drugs were fairly low, indicating that neither activity was a major health life-style component for members of either group.

In contrast to research indicating alcohol consumption to be a common health problem of lesbian women (Diamond & Wilsnack, 1978; Lewis et al., 1982), no statistically significant difference was found between the lesbian and the heterosexual groups in the inclusion or exclusion of alcohol consumption in life-style.

The finding that the heterosexual group had a significantly higher mean for fulfilling family obligations was consistent with the finding that only one lesbian woman in this sample had children. The difference between the lesbian and heterosexual groups in pregnancy history may be reasonably attributed to both age differences and sexual partner preference, especially considering that equivalent percentages of both groups were planning pregnancy in the future. Although the medical community has debated the ethics of providing lesbian women with artificial insemination services (Hanscombe, 1983), support groups and publications have developed within the lesbian community to assist lesbian women in artificial insemination and childbearing (Pies, 1985).

Several results contribute to a perception of a more holistic health orientation among the lesbian women in this sample. The lesbian group reported greater use of alternative diet and meditation/relaxation techniques in their life-styles. Greater participation among the lesbian women in mental health therapy or counseling may reflect greater valuing of introspection and efforts to foster mental and emotional as well as physical well-being. The greater participation of the lesbian group in therapy may also reflect the stress of being lesbian in a heterosexist society in which stigmatization may be the core cultural experience (Stevens & Hall, 1988).

This study is limited by its small, nonprobability, relatively homogenous sample. Further exploration of lesbian women's health life-styles should be carried out with larger, more heterogenous samples. In this study I focused on health life-style activities using a holistic conceptualization of health rather than a narrow gynecological and reproductive focus. As we increase our understanding of lesbian health issues, we would do well to continue to employ this holistic orientation in our research and our clinical practices.

REFERENCES

Diamond, D. L., & Wilsnack, S. C. (1978). Alcohol abuse among lesbians: A descriptive study. *Journal of Homosexuality, 4,* 123–142.

Dritz, S. (1985). Medical aspects of homosexuality. *New England Journal of Medicine, 302,* 463–464.

Good, R. S. (1976). The gynecologist and the lesbian. *Clinical Obstetrics and Gynecology, 19,* 473–482.

Hanscombe, G. (1983). The right to lesbian parenthood. *Journal of Medical Ethics, 9,* 133–135.

Harvey, S. M., Carr, C., & Bernheime, S. (1989). Lesbian mothers: Health care experiences. *Journal of Nurse-Midwifery, 34,* 115–119.

Johnson, S. R., Guenther, S. M., Laube, D. W., & Keettel, W. C. (1981). Factors influencing lesbian gynecologic care: A preliminary study. *American Journal of Obstetrics and Gynecology, 140,* 20–28.

Johnson, S. R., & Palermo, J. L., (1984). Gynecologic care for the lesbian. *Clinical Obstetrics and Gynecology, 27,* 724–731.

Johnson, S. R., Smith, E. M., & Guenther, S. M. (1987). Parenting desires among bisexual women and lesbians. *Journal of Reproductive Medicine, 32*, 198–200.

Lewis, C. E., Saghir, M. T., & Robins, E. (1982). Drinking patterns in homosexual and heterosexual women. *Journal of Clinical Psychiatry, 43*, 277–279.

Olesker, E., & Walsh, L. V. (1984). Childbearing among lesbians: Are we meeting their needs? *Journal of Nurse-Midwifery, 29*, 322–329.

Pies, C. (1985). *Considering parenthood: A workbook for lesbians.* San Francisco: Spinsters Ink.

Robertson, P., & Schacter, J. (1981). Failure to identify venereal disease in a lesbian population. *Sexually Transmitted Disease, 7*, 75–76.

Smith, E. M., Johnson, S. R., & Guenther, S. M. (1985). Health care attitudes and experiences during gynecological care of lesbians and bisexuals. *American Journal of Public Health, 75*, 1085–1087.

Stevens, J. E., & Hall, J. M. (1988). Stigma, health beliefs, and experiences with health care in lesbian women. *Image: Journal of Nursing Scholarship, 20*, 69–73.

Wismont, J. M., & Reame, N. E. (1989). A lesbian childbearing experience: Assisting developmental tasks. *Image: Journal of Nursing Scholarship, 21*, 137–141.

CARING FOR LESBIANS
IN A HOMOPHOBIC SOCIETY

Susan E. Gentry, MSN, ARNP

Division of Maternal-Fetal Medicine, University of Florida, Gainesville, Florida

Lesbians and gays have suffered for centuries from stigmatization by homophobic, heterosexual people in Western society. It is critical for health care providers to have an understanding of alternative life-styles and the unique health concerns of homosexual people in order to provide sensitive and knowledgeable health care. Lesbian health issues such as assessing the sexual orientation of lesbians, parenting issues, lesbian battering, and the older lesbian woman are discussed. My intent in writing this article is to increase the sensitivity, knowledge, and awareness of health care providers caring for lesbians in a homophobic society.

It has been estimated that 1 in 10 females in the United States is lesbian (Kinsey, Pomeroy, Martin, & Gebhard, 1953). This estimate is probably low, because of the stigmatization of homosexual people by Western society (Dworkin & Gutierrez, 1989). Health care providers caring for women will knowingly or unknowingly care for lesbian clients at some point in time. It is critical for health care providers to understand the lesbian life-style and lesbians' unique health concerns in order to become sensitive and knowledgeable about the issues important to lesbian women. In this article I examine homosexuality historically in Western society and discuss health issues currently confronting lesbians as identified in selected literature. My goal is to contribute to the effort to increase health care providers' sensitivity, knowledge, and awareness of the concerns of lesbians in a homophobic society.

HOMOSEXUALITY AND LESBIANISM

According to *Webster's New World Dictionary* (1985), *homosexuality* is "characterized by sexual desire for those of the same sex as oneself,"

The author sincerely thanks Sandra Seymour and Jodi Irving for reviewing this article before its publication.

and *lesbianism* is defined as "homosexuality between women." Believing the term *lesbian* is lacking in depth of meaning, Browning (1984) further defined *lesbian* in the context of a "lesbian identity." Browning's definition encompassed social, emotional, affectional, political, and intellectual issues facing lesbians, as well as their sexual behavior (Zeidenstein, 1990).

In two thirds of the preliterate societies researched worldwide during the 1940s by Ford and Beach, same-sex contact between males was an accepted form of sexual expression (Fogel & Lauver, 1990). However, negative attitudes and homophobia (an irrational fear or hatred of homosexuals and/or lesbians) concerning the practice of homosexuality are frequent in the "civilized world" (Fogel & Lauver, 1990). These negative attitudes are deeply rooted in religious, legal, political, and psychological institutions of Western civilization (Zeidenstein, 1990).

For centuries, identified homosexuals were burned at the stake, hung by the neck, drowned, or beheaded (Zeidenstein, 1990). Homosexuals discovered in Nazi concentration camps during World War II were forced to wear pink triangles, and hundreds of thousands of homosexuals and lesbians were massacred (Browning, 1984). Some religious institutions, such as the Catholic and Jewish faiths, have denounced homosexuality as sinful, and some Presbyterian and other Protestant leaders have declared that same-sex sexual practices appear to be against the laws of God and nature (Fogel & Lauver, 1990).

Until 1973, homosexuality was classified as a mental illness by the American Psychiatric Association (Gillow & Davis, 1987). Successful treatment of this "disease" was believed to be changing the client from a homosexual to a heterosexual orientation. Methods such as confrontation, subtle persuasion, exploration of childhood trauma, and even electroshock were used as treatment regimens by psychiatrists (Markowitz, 1991; Sang, 1989). These behavioral and aversive therapies were used in spite of the mounting evidence indicating that homosexuality was not pathological.

In 1973, the American Psychiatric Association declassified homosexuality as a mental illness in the *Diagnostic and Statistical Manual of Mental Disorders,* except for those people who were in conflict with their orientation (Dworkin & Gutierrez, 1989). This was the beginning of a movement to end the endorsed prejudice of mental health professionals and others toward homosexuals and lesbians.

In spite of this proclaimed dissociation of homosexuality and mental illness by the American Psychiatric Association, many homosexual and lesbian clients still feel that heterosexual psychologists and psychiatrists suggest that the homosexual life-style is less than normal or less preferable than being heterosexual (Markowitz, 1991). Understandably, they tend to seek out gay and lesbian mental health counselors (McDermott, Tyndall, & Lichtenberg, 1989).

Further, Randall's (1989) study of 100 faculty members of a midwestern nursing college indicated that more than half of the faculty believed lesbianism is an unnatural expression of human sexuality. Seventeen percent of the sample indicated they thought lesbians would molest children. Twenty-eight percent of the nursing faculty reported they would have difficulty conversing with a known lesbian. Randall suggested that this difficulty in communication would affect the quality of education offered to nursing students and set a precedent for continued misunderstanding of lesbians and their life-styles. Until health care providers, and particularly health care educators, examine their own views and values about sexuality and internalized homophobia, they will be unable to provide the humanistic, nonjudgmental, and sensitive care gay and lesbian clients have the right to expect.

COMING-OUT ISSUES

Coming out was defined by Deevy (1990) and Gillow and Davis (1987) as disclosing one's homosexuality by recognizing, acknowledging, and/or acting on one's sexual orientation. The term is also used metaphorically to describe stepping out of a "closet." In psychology, a "closet" is a figure of speech that refers to an emotional hiding place where one does not have to disclose one's true identity (Zeidenstein, 1990). To come out risks stepping out of a place believed to be safe, both physically and emotionally.

Zeidenstein (1990) found in her study of 20 lesbians that the fear and unpleasantness of coming out influenced the majority of her subjects to postpone their gynecological care or to seek lesbian-sensitive health care providers. Many of the women in Zeidenstein's study who did choose to come out did so to dispute the health care provider's negating heterosexual assumptions, such as assuming the client had a need for birth control or that the sexual partner of the client was male.

The risks or fears of coming out to health care providers identified by Smith, Heaton, and Seiver (1990) were many. Included were the fear that health care will be withheld or substandard, the fear of rejection by the health care provider, and the fear that the health care provider will moralize to the client or try to change her sexual orientation. Moreover, many lesbians fear that the health care provider will violate their trust and confidentiality.

There are many risks to homosexuals coming out in society as well. By disclosing their homosexuality, lesbians may experience rejection, shame, and humiliation from family members and friends who do not understand the homosexual life-style (Gillow & Davis, 1987). Lesbians may also experience stress as a result of societal norms and laws against homosexuality related to sexual practices (Loulan, 1988) and lesbian parenting (Gillow & Davis, 1987). Not only has there been employment and housing discrimination against gays and lesbians, but homosexuals are at times confronted with physical violence and antigay rhetoric (Zeidenstein, 1990). Gay-bashing is commonplace in high schools throughout the United States, prompting young adolescents to remain closeted for their own survival (Coleman & Remafedi, 1989; Hersch, 1991).

LESBIAN HEALTH ISSUES

Assessing the Sexual Orientation of Lesbians

Information about a client's sexual orientation is an important component of the health history (Smith et al., 1990). How the client is approached during the health history taking may assist with this disclosure. One group of lesbian women preferred to be asked directly about their sexual orientation (Smith et al., 1990). Other lesbians choose to come out on their health history questionnaires by answering heterosexual-assuming questions with further explanations. For example, their response to the question "Are you sexually active?" might be, "Yes, with a woman" (Zeidenstein, 1990). Other lesbians feel they are identifiable without verbally coming out by the symbolic buttons or jewelry depicting a lesbian orientation (e.g., a double female symbol; a pink triangle; or a labyrus, an ancient matriarchal symbol of female power) they wear. Others feel they are recognized merely by having an androgynous appearance (Zeidenstein, 1990).

Some lesbians have suggested that health care providers need to be sensitive to alternative sexual orientations by including the categories of "lesbian," "bisexual," "celibate," and "homosexual," as well as a category for "committed relationship" or "gay/lesbian couple" on the marital status portion of the health history form (Zeidenstein, 1990).

Recently, some psychologists have written that if a lesbian client discloses her sexual orientation, it is important for health care providers to be "lesbian affirmative" in their interactions (Loulan, 1988; Murphy, 1989). It is not enough for health care providers to passively accept the lesbian life-style of a client; they must actively validate the client's sexual orientation by recognizing both the challenges and strengths of lesbian relationships. The health care provider's nonjudgmental acknowledgment of the client's sexual orientation may help the client to develop a more positive self-image and recover from the damage of negative stigmatization and homophobia that has occurred during her life and continues to occur in Western society (Murphy, 1989). Confirmation and validation of the client's sexual orientation by her health care provider also encourage a caring, open, and trusting relationship between client and provider, facilitating optimum health promotion and wellness.

If a client makes the decision to disclose her sexual orientation to the provider, the provider needs to be sensitive about charting this information. In one study, one fourth of the lesbians questioned said they would not come out to their health care provider if their sexual orientation would be recorded on their medical records (Zeidenstein, 1990). In light of the discrimination and persecution suffered by gays and lesbians, the provider should always seek permission from the client before charting this information on the medical record. The health care provider should also assess the importance of or the need for charting such information.

Lesbians, Human Immunodeficiency Virus Infection, and Sexually Transmitted Diseases

Many false assumptions have been made about lesbians and human immunodeficiency virus infection. Because HIV has been labeled in the United States a disease of homosexuals and intravenous drug abusers, many people wrongly consider lesbians a high-risk group. According to the Centers for Disease Control (1990), lesbians as a group are at very low risk for developing HIV. However, it is still very important that health care providers continue to educate lesbians concerning safer sex practices, as women in general are at increasingly greater risk for HIV infection.

The prevalence of vaginal infections and sexually transmitted diseases (STDs) is also low among lesbians (Zeidenstein, 1990). However, if a lesbian presents with an STD or vaginal infection, misinformation concerning the treatment of her sexual partner is often given, such as "Have your partner use condoms while you are being treated for this infection" (assuming the partner is male). By initially assessing the client's sexual relationship, the health care provider can provide more accurate information to the client.

Lesbians and Parenting

In their study of lesbian mothers, Harvey, Carr, and Bernheine (1989) found that a majority of lesbians not only want to parent, but also want to experience pregnancy and childbirth. Some lesbian parenting options include artificial insemination from a known or unknown donor, adoption, and heterosexual intercourse (Smith et al., 1990).

Artificial insemination can be performed in an outpatient women's clinic, an infertility clinic, an obstetrician/gynecologist's office, or the home. Sperm can come from a sperm bank or a male friend or lover. Because of the possible transmission of HIV from unscreened donor sperm, as well as potential legal custody battles, more lesbians are turning to sperm banks for donor sperm (Zeidenstein, 1990). The choice of the method of insemination raises significant legal custody issues, especially in the case of a known donor (Smith et al., 1990). The lesbian client who desires to parent should be advised to seek counsel with a local legal practitioner or to call the Lesbian Mothers National Defense Fund in Seattle, Washington, at (206) 325-2643, to obtain a national referral list of attorneys who specialize in homosexual and lesbian parenting issues (Smith et al., 1990).

Adoption is a limited alternative for lesbians in Western society today, because adoption agencies generally refuse to accept adoptive parents outside of a heterosexual marriage. In the case of a lesbian woman who desires to adopt the children of her partner, because many courts view lesbianism unfavorably, it is likely that the adoption would be denied. Also, same-sex marriages are unrecognized by law in the United States; therefore unless a lesbian woman presents herself as a single individual who desires to adopt a baby, adoption may not be the most realistic option available to the lesbian couple (Smith et al., 1990).

Lesbian Battering and Partner Abuse

If it has been difficult for lesbian women to disclose their sexual orientation to their health care providers, one can imagine their silence concerning lesbian battering. There is the myth among lesbians that all lesbian relationships are exclusively passionate, loving, and, above all, never violent (Morrow & Hawxhurst, 1989). The fear of dispelling the myth of the ideal relationship reinforces the silence of the lesbian victim of battering.

Lesbian victims of partner abuse are even less likely than their heterosexual counterparts to seek help in shelters or from counselors (Morrow & Hawxhurst, 1989). For this reason, the health care provider must be extremely sensitive to the possibility of a client's involvement in a battering relationship. Lesbian battering can come in many forms: physical assaults, sexual assaults, emotional threats, psychological abuse, economic control, and homophobic control, to name a few. Homophobic control involves threatening to tell family, friends, employer, or others that the victim is a lesbian, when disclosure of that information would be devastating to the victim (Brand & Kidd, 1986).

If a health care provider knows or suspects that lesbian battering is occurring, the provider should encourage the client to seek help. Becoming informed about the local lesbian network of lesbian-sensitive mental health counselors and support groups is helpful when making referrals for a client.

Older Lesbian Women

Older lesbian women are at the greatest risk for unmet health needs, because of their "triple minority status" of old age, female gender, and alternative sexual orientation (Deevy, 1990, p. 35). Further, older lesbian women may be deeply closeted or especially secretive about their sexual orientation, because they grew up before the time of the Gay Liberation Movement. During the 1940s and 1950s, exposure of one's homosexuality almost guaranteed loss of family, jobs, and basic security (Deevy, 1990).

Health care providers may not be sensitive to subtle clues to the older lesbian's sexual orientation, such as having the same female roommate for 35 years. Also, older lesbian women often refer to themselves indirectly as "people like us" rather than using the term *lesbian,* and prefer not to be labeled by others, including researchers (Deevy, 1990).

Communication is difficult if the health care provider routinely assumes heterosexuality in female clients and the older lesbian woman is deeply closeted. As a first step, health care providers need to face their own prejudices and develop sensitivity to the possibility that an older woman may be a lesbian. It is also important to be respectful of the client's relationship with her significant other. Old age is a period in which interdependency on traditional and nontraditional family support systems is vital for the maintenance and promotion of wellness.

CONCLUSION

Health care providers must confront their own feelings, prejudices, and beliefs regarding human sexuality and alternative life-styles in order to provide optimal health care to varied clients. Lesbians will turn to their health care providers for information about health care issues, and it is important that the health care provider communicates understanding of these issues and makes appropriate referrals.

REFERENCES

Brand, T., & Kidd, A. (1986). Frequency of physical aggression in heterosexual and female homosexual dyads. *Psychology Reports, 59,* 1307–1313.

Browning, C. (1984). Changing theories of lesbianism: Challenging the stereotypes. In T. Darty & S. Potter (Eds.), *Women-Identified Women*. Palo Alto, CA: Mayfield.

Centers for Disease Control. (1990, June). National AIDS Information Clearinghouse, telephone (800) 458-5231. *Statement on Female-to-Female Transmission of HIV*, issued June 1990. (Statment read over telephone by a representative of the National AIDS Information Clearinghouse.)

Coleman, E., & Remafedi, G. (1989). Gay, lesbian, and bisexual adolescents: A critical challenge to counselors. *Journal of Counseling and Development, 68*, 36–40.

Deevy, S. (1990). Older lesbian women: An invisible minority. *Journal of Gerontological Nursing, 16*(5), 37–39.

Dworkin, S. H., & Gutierrez, F. (1989). Counselors be aware clients come in every size, shape, color, and sexual orientation. *Journal of Counseling and Development, 68*, 6–10.

Fogel, C. I., & Lauver, D. (1990). *Sexual health promotion*. Philadelphia: W. B. Saunders.

Gillow, K. E., & Davis, L. L. (1987). Lesbian stress and coping methods. *Journal of Psychosocial Nursing, 25*(9), 28–32.

Harvey, S. M., Carr, C., & Bernheine, S. (1989). Lesbian mothers' health care experiences. *Journal of Nurse-Midwifery, 34*(3), 115–119.

Hersch, P. (1991). Secret lives. Gays and lesbians in therapy. *The Family Therapy Networker, 15*(1), 36–43.

Kinsey, A. C., Pomeroy, W. B., Martin, C. E., & Gebhard, P. H. (1953). *Sexual behavior in the human female*. Philadelphia: W. B. Saunders.

Loulan, J. A. (1988). Research on the sex practices of 1,566 lesbians and the clinical applications. *Women and Therapy: A Feminist Quarterly, 7*(23), 221–234.

Markowitz, L. M. (1991). Homosexuality: Are we still in the dark? *The Family Therapy Networker, 15*(1), 26–35.

McDermott, D., Tyndall, L., & Lichtenberg, J. (1989). Factors related to counselor preference among gays and lesbians. *Journal of Counseling and Development, 68*, 31–35.

Morrow, S. K., & Hawxhurst, D. M. (1989). Lesbian partner abuse: Implications for therapists. *Journal of Counseling and Development, 68*, 58–62.

Murphy, B. C. (1989). Lesbian couples and their parents: The effects of perceived parental attitudes on the couple. *Journal of Counseling and Development, 68*, 46–51.

Randall, C. E. (1989). Lesbian phobia among BSN educators: A survey. *Journal of Nursing Education, 28*, 302–306.

Sang, B. E. (1989). New directions in lesbian research, theory, and education. *Journal of Counseling and Development, 68*, 92–96.

Smith, M., Heaton, C., & Seiver, D. (1990). Health concerns of lesbians. *Physician Assistant, 14*(1), 81–94.

Webster's New World Dictionary. (1985). Springfield, MA: Merriam-Webster.

Zeidenstein, L. (1990). Gynecological and childbearing needs of lesbians. *Journal of Nurse-Midwifery, 35*(1), 10–16.

AN EXPLORATION OF LESBIANS' IMAGES
OF RECOVERY FROM ALCOHOL PROBLEMS

Joanne M. Hall, RN, MA

Department of Mental Health, Community, and Administrative Nursing
School of Nursing, University of California, San Francisco

The author's purposes in this article are to explore the images lesbians use to describe their recovery from alcohol problems and to derive from this exercise relevant implications for health care. Lesbians' experiences in recovery are particularly significant because of growing concerns about the prevalence of alcohol problems among lesbians, the vulnerability of lesbians as an aggregate, and the cultural trend away from substance use in lesbian communities. Images of recovery are the descriptions that people offer about their healing from alcohol problems. They are the frameworks by which problem drinkers interpret the meanings of their experiences and determine which aspects of their lives are most pertinent to their recovery efforts. The images persons use to represent their progress and the difficulties they encounter in recovery also provide important bases for developing relevant resources, therapeutic techniques, and social support. Excerpts from an ongoing ethnographic interview study about the recovery experiences of lesbians with alcohol problems illustrate the diversity of recovery images that are characteristic of this population.

Lesbians' experiences in recovery from alcohol problems are of interest to health care providers because of growing concern about the prevalence of alcohol problems among lesbians, the established vulnerability of lesbians as an aggregate, and the recent cultural trend away from substance use in lesbian communities. In this article, I establish the significance of lesbians' alcohol problems and explore the images lesbians use to describe their recovery from alcohol problems. Examples of lesbians' descriptions of their recovery are taken from an ongoing ethno-

Joanne M. Hall is a PhD candidate at the University of California, San Francisco.

graphic interview study on the help-seeking and recovery experiences of
lesbians with alcohol problems. Insights from these images are then
used to derive relevant implications for health care.

Researchers, clinicians, and lesbians themselves believe that substance abuse problems among lesbians are more prevalent and more
severe than those seen in the general population (Burke, 1982; Cantu,
1985; Fifield, Latham, & Phillips, 1977; Hastings, 1982; Hepburn &
Gutierrez, 1988; McKirnan & Peterson, 1989a, 1989b; McNally, 1989;
Morales & Graves, 1983; Nicoloff & Stiglitz, 1987; Saghir & Robins,
1973; Schilit, Clark, & Shallenberger, 1988; Stevens & Hall, 1988;
Weathers, 1976). Skepticism is appropriate in interpreting prevalence
rates of alcohol problems among lesbians, however, because accurate
estimates are not obtainable in this largely hidden, stigmatized group
(Morin, 1977; Nardi, 1982). In the only available study (Bradford &
Ryan, 1988) based on a national, convenience sample of lesbians ($N =$
1,917), 25% of lesbians reported drinking several times a week and 6%
reported drinking daily. Fourteen percent of the sample reported being
worried about their substance use, and 16% had sought help for alcohol
or drug problems in the past. These figures provide evidence that lesbians may be both susceptible to alcohol problems and prone to self-
criticism regarding their use of alcohol.

Lesbians are an important source of information about alcohol use
and recovery patterns because of the particular social and political vul-
nerabilities they experience. Lesbians have been frequently overlooked
and/or pathologized in research and clinical endeavors (Stevens & Hall,
1991). Substance abuse in women is highly stigmatized. To be a lesbian
problem drinker entails additional stigmatization, which may pose difficulties in recognizing the problem, feeling safe in seeking health care,
and maintaining a positive self-image in the recovery process (Hall,
1990a, 1990b; Johnson & Palermo, 1984; Stevens & Hall, 1988; Szasz,
1970; Ziebold, 1979).

Lesbians seem to be on the cutting edge of a generalized cultural
trend away from substance use (Room, 1988). Lesbian communities
have been engaged in dialogue about alcohol use and recovery from
alcohol problems for the past several decades. Lesbians' association of
substance use with internalized oppression, sexism, and the ghettoiza-
tion of lesbians in the bar subculture has contributed to this movement
(Hall, 1991). Twelve Step and other mutual- and self-help programs can
be viewed as meeting important social needs within lesbian communities, often replacing those formerly met by the lesbian bar subculture.
These include the needs for affiliation, privacy, safety, socialization, and
spiritual expression (Hall, 1991; Herman, 1988).

Why are images of recovery important? The ways in which problem drinkers conceptualize recovery serve as frameworks for interpreting the meaning of their experiences and determining which aspects of life are salient to their recovery efforts. Images of recovery are the descriptions that people offer about their healing from alcohol problems. These images may be metaphorical. They may communicate the totality of the experience or only particular features. The images persons use to represent their progress and the difficulties they encounter in recovery provide important bases for developing relevant resources, therapeutic techniques, and social support. Individuals may use a single image of recovery, or they may describe a repertoire of images, each representing a particular aspect or period of recovery. The potential clinical value that images of recovery hold in terms of revealing individual and collective meanings about recovery indicates that much more information is needed about the sources, variety, and uses of these images in recovering populations.

In the ongoing ethnographic interview study of which this analysis is a part, 35 lesbians in recovery from alcohol problems living in the San Francisco Bay Area were interviewed during 1990 and 1991. Sixty-eight percent of the participants were Euro-Americans, 17% African-Americans, 9% Latinas, 3% Asian-Americans, and 3% Native Americans. Participants' ages ranged from 24 to 54 years, with a mean of 37. The socioeconomic backgrounds of participants were as follows: 46% were working class, 31% were middle class, and 23% were impoverished. Their years of education varied from 12 to 22 years, with a mean of 16. All 35 women reported abusing alcohol; 91% reported they had abused other drugs as well. Many also reported difficulties with other compulsive behaviors concerning food (34%), "codependency" (23%), sexual activity (11%), or money (6%). Length of time in recovery was self-reported and ranged from 1 to 25 years, with a mean of 6. Seventy-four percent of the participants were actively involved in Alcoholics Anonymous (AA), and the 26% who did not participate in AA were at least familiar with the AA program format through literature, prior involvement, or the influence of friends.

The term *alcohol problems* is used herein to avoid the limitations of the narrower, traditional disease model, signified by the term *alcoholism*. Abstinence from alcohol and other drugs, although not the sole focus, is considered to be a sound foundation for recovery. However, the occurrence of relapses is recognized as potentially meaningful in facilitating positive transitions in recovery for some individuals (Hall, 1990b). The term *recovery* has historically been used in health care to designate the period and process of restoration after illness or injury. This definition carries the implication that recovery is a process that ends or is completed within a specific, if variable, period. *Recuperation* and *rehabilitation* are related terms reflecting this temporally limited quality. The medical notion of recovery is primarily focused on physical and mental changes that move the individual away from the illness condition, such that recovery can be measured according to the presence or absence of symptoms of pathology or trauma. In terms of alcohol problems, recovery has a more complex set of dimensions, dimensions that go beyond the disappearance of symptoms to include behavioral, social, and cultural considerations (Tomko, 1988). In the following section, notions of recovery represented in AA, a major cultural source of recovery imagery, are explored as a point of comparison for the images lesbians described in the interviews.

AA AS A SOURCE OF CULTURAL MEANING FOR RECOVERY

The concept of "alcoholism" as a disease entity was advanced by medicine to counter the idea that alcohol overuse was simply a matter of moral weakness. AA, perhaps the most important source of cultural meaning regarding alcohol problems, was formally established in 1935 by a group of self-defined "alcoholics" who found a way to abstain from alcohol and improve the quality of their lives through group identification and the Twelve Steps that they followed in the process (Kurtz, 1988). AA rhetoric has it that "alcoholism" is similar to an "allergy" to alcohol that renders the "alcoholic" physiologically incapable of drinking in a reasonable manner. It also describes the problem as being "powerless over alcohol," with the result that one's life becomes "unmanageable" (Alcoholics Anonymous World Services, 1976). The term for recovery initially used by AA, and the term that dominates its literature, is *sobriety* (Alcoholics Anonymous World Services, 1976). Sobriety has two basic aspects: abstinence from alcohol and other mind-altering substances not medically sanctioned and continued improvement of one's social and spiritual relations through practice of AA's Twelve Steps.

The term *recovery* has gained currency as an increasing number of aspects of life have become associated with the healing process in the experience of recovering persons and groups. Recovery is therefore an evolving concept (Tomko, 1988). Some persons with alcohol problems integrate the idea of sobriety with the processes involved in addressing other, non-alcohol-related compulsive problems they face. An ever-increasing number of Twelve Step programs have been based on the AA model, such as Narcotics Anonymous, Gamblers Anonymous, Overeaters Anonymous, and Cocaine Anonymous. The Twelve Step model has even been adapted for nonaddictive problems, as in the case of Incest Survivors Anonymous.

The AA view, which has contributed heavily to predominant mainstream views of alcohol problems, combines moral and spiritual difficulties related to excessive drinking with the medical profession's disease notion of "alcoholism" (Earle, 1982; Jellinek, 1960; Levine, 1984; Peele, 1986; Shaffer, 1986). Rather than a radical departure from the moralistic discourse of the temperance movement, AA can be viewed as a transformation of this discourse, preserving some of the moral overtones surrounding alcohol problems (Levine, 1984; Royce, 1986). The obvious Christian imagery and terminology used in AA writings is illustrative of this. AA's dual focus on "alcoholism" as both a disease and a cause for "defects of character" relieves addictive drinkers of guilt for having the problem while holding them accountable to do something constructive about it.

The primary image of recovery in AA is one of conversion. The conversion image of recovery has three general phases or dimensions, which are reflected in the format of telling one's story in AA: What it was like, what happened, and what it is like now (Maxwell, 1984; Rudy, 1986; Thune, 1977). In religious terms this might be expressed as sin or moral decline, transformation, and then moral virtuousness. This image of recovery is one of unidirectional change from negativity to positivity. As in the notion of being "born again," conversion implies the creation of a new person and the abandonment of old ways of living. Contrasting terms such as *lost/found, condemned/saved,* and *drunk/sober* reflect the unidirectional change seen in the conversion image. Classically, conversion is conceptualized as a once-in-a-lifetime occurrence (James, 1902/1961). However, clinical experience reveals that a once-and-for-all transition from problem drinking to continual abstinence is the exception rather than the rule. This is corroborated by references in AA literature to "slips" or relapses, which are not uncommon (Alcoholics Anonymous World Services, 1976).

LESBIANS' IMAGES OF RECOVERY

Conversion is one image lesbians use to describe their recovery experiences. But conversion alone is inadequate to describe all the experiences lesbians have in recovery. In the following sections various alternative images of recovery expressed by lesbians are described, and examples of each are provided in the form of quotes from the ethnographic interviews. Although these examples may seem to suggest that each woman had only one view of recovery, in most cases a number of images were reported. Images varied depending on the temporal period of recovery being described and which specific issues or conflicts were being addressed. In other words, a repertoire of images was ordinarily used to express the meaning of recovery.

Recovery as Physical Transition

Some participants emphasized physical changes, improvements, or awarenesses as exemplifying what recovery meant to them. These images were most often used in discussing early recovery (the first year or two). Themes about physical transitions included increased perception of health and illness phenomena, initiation of more appropriate exercise and daily living habits, and taking responsibility for pre-existing chronic illnesses.

When I stopped drinking, and I was a daily drinker, I got one virus after another for a year. My immune system must have been in shambles from the damage I had done. It wasn't like I was just getting sick in recovery, but that only without the alcohol was I really aware of just how physically messed up my addiction had made me.

I didn't deal with emotions or anything for the first year. I had to learn how to physically live, and that meant learning to make my bed every day, shower, eat. And that was all I could do. I rarely left my house.

The doctors told me I had liver damage. It took a long time for it to sink in what that meant. It was serious. And when I was drunk and stoned I never took care of my diabetes. A big thing in my recovery is that I show up for the appointments, I follow my food plan, and I have to be responsible for my illness. I already have neuropathies. But I can regulate the diabetes now so those things don't get worse. I can't go back and do it over, I have to look ahead.

Recovery as Personal Growth

Some lesbians referred to recovery as a journey of personal growth and spiritual development. They recalled various phases in this journey, which were characterized by specific focal issues. Among these issues were isolation, self-centeredness, judgmentalness, lack of belief in a power greater than themselves, willfulness, dishonesty, and grief. For these women, abstinence from alcohol and other drugs was a prerequisite to the journey, but not the journey itself. They reported that progress in the journey was marked by increases in serenity, that is, self-acceptance, wisdom, and inner peace. Most of these women were involved in AA, which is reflected in their choice of language. Often these women would say that recovery was, for them, an "inside job."

> It's about growth, it's a stretch. . . . I don't isolate now. I don't want to judge people. I don't gossip. . . . I haven't had major awakenings but gradually I have changed. . . . I couldn't do this without the AA program.

> I had a great deal of guilt. I would tell everybody everything, compulsively. It was overexposure. I had to stop doing that because it was really like beating myself up all the time. I was still atoning for sins or something.

> I used to be self-centered, egotistical, omnipotent, but under that was pure fear. I dealt with fear by showing anger or rage. I was this mean cobra. I can own my fears now, and I don't have to convince myself of being superhuman, like I am beyond such primal emotions.

Recovery as Struggle with Compulsivity

Patterns of recovery from alcohol problems for many women, including lesbians, are related to and interwoven with the course of recovery for similar problems, such as eating disorders, overspending, smoking, or codependency (Hepburn & Gutierrez, 1988; Tomko, 1988; Wilson-Schaef, 1987). Many of the lesbians interviewed described having several addictive problems. Alcohol abuse was seen as only one symptom of a larger, often nameless life disturbance characterized by compulsivity. Other drug abuse, overeating, anorexia, overspending, sex addiction, and codependency (focusing excessively on others' needs) were some of these concurrent problems. For these women, recovery was a serial or simultaneous struggle with one or more of these compulsive syndromes, for which similar strategies were applied. Twelve Step programs such as Narcotics Anonymous, Overeaters Anonymous, Sex and Love Addicts Anonymous, Debtors Anonymous, and Codependents Anonymous were typically used. For these women, approaches to recovery that included all of their compulsive tendencies were valued. Involvement in AA could be problematic if concurrent problems were deemed unimportant or unrelated by fellow AA members. These women also battled a sense of fragmentation fostered by health services that specialize in only one compulsive behavior.

> My strongest conviction says that the professionals shouldn't discount the power of food, that addiction. Don't belittle it. Cross addiction and poly-addiction are real, and it could be lots of things—gambling for instance. You have to treat all these things across the gamut because they all can kill

you. Also, we don't all fit the "stages" that are in the books, so you should keep the doors open for different experiences.

I did some work on codependency after I stopped drinking. I depended on therapeutic support groups and went to AA only periodically. From the fourth year on I have had a lot of money problems. I have lots of debts from that. And the alcohol and my eating disorder were very much related. I was always aware that alcohol had calories. To keep my weight I'd fast all day so I could give myself permission to drink. . . . The speed allowed me not to eat. I hope to get to the place where the self-hatred and shame go away, because they tie in with the alcohol and the weight thing.

Recovery as Reclaiming the Self

Some lesbians reported that their alcohol and drug use were symptoms of underlying, unresolved trauma from the past. They found that when they stopped using alcohol and other drugs, they began to experience the emergence of memories and feelings that had been denied or dissociated from painful prior, usually childhood, events, such as rape, incest, battering, and/or neglect. As memories were recovered and feelings named, these women believed that they were literally retrieving and restoring parts of themselves. They often used individual and group therapy, art therapy, and other nonmedical means of understanding their own responses to the trauma as well as to explore family-of-origin dynamics. This work was often kept separate from AA involvement, and in some cases AA was seen as not fully sensitive to the impact of these family and trauma issues for women. For instance, AA advocates forgiveness as a core element of recovery. Many of these women did not feel it was appropriate to forgive the perpetrators of their abuse. The work of reclaiming the past can be problematic in some AA environments. Some lesbian interviewees, for whom the issues of childhood trauma were not pertinent or not currently relevant, perceived the discussion of family-of-origin dynamics and childhood abuse as straying from the focus of AA, which they deemed to be abstinence from alcohol and working the Twelve Steps.

The problem with AA is that they take out the newcomer's brain at the door and insert the Twelve Steps. How can you really recover, how can you learn about yourself? What happened to me as a kid has everything to do with who I am now.

The slip I had when I was sober two months was about sexual abuse, incest. My therapist had said, "Have you considered that you may have been raped in the past?" The next two days I had intense self-hatred, and

I knew she was right even though I had no memories yet. . . . My sponsor didn't get it, so I accused her of not giving a damn about me and immediately got drunk. . . . But after three days I started back, because I knew I had to deal with this in sobriety.

I got really scared at a group meeting and started remembering childhood things. . . . I went out of my body, everything was in slow motion. This lasted five days, where I was helpless and a friend had to take care of me. . . . But I realized I had survived this pain without a drink. . . . For me it was feeling responsible for my whole family, feeling I didn't help them, didn't measure up. . . . and there was physical abuse, threats. . . . I'd have these out-of-body experiences whenever I had a crisis, and my emotions were becoming flat. I had big black gaps in my memory, I mean before I ever used drugs or alcohol. . . . I realize now that I wasn't a horrible, inadequate person, but that there was this stuff that had happened to me, and that the effects were reversible.

Recovery as Connection/Reconnection

Isolation and a feeling of being alien in the universe are common experiences for those with alcohol problems. It is not clear which occurs first, the feeling of being "outside" or the alcohol abuse. For many of the women, being lesbian was a strong basis for feeling like an outsider, a feeling that often plagued them from adolescence on. Recovery was presented by many of those interviewed as a process of finding meaningful connections with others like themselves and of opening up to the possibilities of new relationships.

Connecting with other women, and especially with lesbians, became a key part of their recovery. They often described being unable to accept fully the idea of being lesbian in a positive way before they stopped drinking and using drugs. Many referred to Living Sober, an annual lesbian/gay AA gathering in San Francisco, as a turning point in their connection or reconnection with the recovering lesbian community. Likewise, some of the African-American and Latina women interviewed described recovery as a process of accepting their racial and ethnic heritages and confronting painful racial conflicts that they had buried through their substance use. Choosing which AA meetings to attend reflects the need to connect with others "like me," although the basis for such identification changes during different periods of recovery (Vourakis, 1989). Some lesbians chose to attend lesbian AA meetings, but many others reported feeling out of place or intimidated even in these meetings. The milieu of comfort in AA tended to change over time for individuals, depending on their needs. General mainstream AA meetings or those specifically for people of color, women, atheists, etc., were examples of meetings chosen to meet specific needs for connectedness.

> You get this higher power connection when you realize that to sit with someone, really be with them, is a spiritual experience. . . . There's something powerful about being in a room full of people who have something in common. . . . I'm bigger than what's in here, in this body of mine.

> I go to all lesbian meetings now. I have to be able to be myself, to feel safe. This wasn't a big deal for me at first, because then I just wanted to get by one day without drinking or using dope.

> I go to straight AA meetings. . . . I think it is a chance for me to learn tolerance, and for me to teach them tolerance about gay people. It's a way of connecting with other parts of the world I would never have before recovery.

> I think the AA Big Book has historical significance. . . . I like to see myself as a part of that tradition going all the way back to the beginning of AA.

> It's about comfort levels. Some lesbians can't deal with all-lesbian meetings, and some people of color can't start out at the people of color meetings. You know, it can feel too close to home. . . . It shouldn't be assumed where someone will feel comfortable. Sometimes you connect with the most unlikely people.

> I used to think as an adolescent that one of these days I'd be white. Even cocaine was a way of disconnecting from the blackness, the black community. . . . Black-on-black crime disgusted me. . . . All my life my education was all about proving to me that I am not black. After two years in recovery I can say education is for education's sake.

Recovery as Cyclical/Celebratory

Recovery was characterized by some women as a temporal, cyclical process, often highlighted by celebration and commemoration. These temporal markers of recovery included both positive and negative events, such as detoxification, AA "birthdays" (anniversaries of sobriety dates), commonly designated "difficult periods" in sobriety, the timing and precipitants of relapses, the attachment to people who entered recovery at the same time as oneself, annual AA conferences such as Living Sober, and the celebration of holidays in a "clean and sober" state. This image of recovery was also reflected in statements about the need for predictability in recovery. Individuals sought knowledge about recovery as a universal experience and tried to develop insight into their own individual rhythms wherein similar issues re-emerged in a cyclical fashion throughout recovery.

> I always remember the women who got into recovery the same time I did, especially each year when we celebrate our sobriety date together. I grieve for the ones who are not in recovery any longer. . . . And then every year there is Living Sober when for five days I am intensely immersed into the issues and victories of my recovery.

> Lately I feel overwhelmed, with my birthday coming up. You know I was really sick. Really sick. I guess I feel pretty grateful. Getting in touch with the goddess and my own feminine aspects, my cycles, was like coming home for me. I began to study and do rituals.

> When I was sober 2 years I had a weird experience, which changed everything. It was a ceremony, called a "spiritual cleansing." This ritual loosened me up so that I could access my memories of my childhood and be present emotionally like never before. The compulsion to drink left me. . . . I hardly ever talk about this, except in general terms. My friend says she doesn't know what it was all about, but it sure worked.

Recovery as Vocational Change

Many of those interviewed made decisions in their early recovery to return to school or change careers. They saw recovery as an opportunity and perhaps a duty to contribute to society through their work. Often they chose helping fields such as nursing, counseling, and social work. Of course, these are also among the occupations most open to women in general. Significantly, many chose to specialize in substance abuse work. They described how they are encouraged to continue their own recovery by firsthand observation of the ravages of addiction that they encounter in their work.

> When I was using drugs and booze, I was doing the corporate ladder climb; everything on the outside looked good. . . . but I hated my life, I didn't know how to live my life. . . . So in recovery I just dropped out of that. I am in school to study massage and holistic healing techniques.

> I was a client in a newly formed, nonprofessional gay/lesbian treatment program on the East Coast. . . . What they had to say rang true for me. . . . I ended up as an alumni, then a staff member, and eventually an administrator of this program. I had a degree in psychology, but I was hired more for my recovery experience.

Recovery as Empowerment

For many, alcohol abuse was seen as a product of an addictive, racist, patriarchal society, and therefore recovery was viewed as a process of personal and collective empowerment as women, sometimes as women of color, and as lesbians. AA was viewed negatively by some, but not all, of these women because it retains the trappings of white, male, Christian, middle-class culture and recommends that the person with an alcohol problem surrender his or her will. This seemed incongruous to many interviewees because of their perception that most women, lesbians in particular, have felt powerless for much of their lives. An empowerment image of recovery encouraged them to take control, to be critical, and to trust their own instincts. Further, they gained the insight that issues of addiction should not be separated from the politics of race, class, gender, disability, sexual orientation, and age.

> I got married very young and it didn't work. I used to think, when I was still drinking, "What's wrong with me?" Now I think, "What's wrong with the setup?"

> "Recovery" isn't the way I define my whole existence any more, like I did in the beginning. Now the daily problems I face are due to being a woman in a misogynist culture and a lesbian in a homophobic culture.

> AA needs to get out of the patriarchy and incorporate blacks and women, lesbians more. . . . This stuff didn't matter to me when I first came into the program.

> I still hate the Lord's Prayer and I refuse to say it at AA meetings. The Christian flavor of AA is insulting to me as a lesbian.

> As a Latina I have a lot of issues around race and culture and living in the U.S. that I have not really resolved yet in sobriety. But I know these are the issues which can make me relapse. And I have a real hard time with sexual abuse, which is so active in the ghettos and barrios. . . . And it's not a multicultural lesbian community yet. We have to deal with the reality of our oppression in recovery.

Recovery as Social Transition

Lesbian bars have traditionally been centers for socialization, where friendships and affectional relationships can form and where lesbians can be themselves, away from societal scrutiny and prejudice. These bars have also served a stigmatized community's collective needs for family, church, affiliation, and protection from violence. To leave the bar scene therefore presents a threat to many lesbians that is not paralleled in the experiences of straight people in recovery (Hall, 1991). For this reason, recovery becomes for many lesbians a process of rebuilding a social network that is not centered around alcohol use and lesbian bars. In recent years, Twelve Step groups have become more acceptable among lesbians as collectively they have moved away from substance use, particularly in urban coastal regions. Gradually, where available, lesbian and lesbian/gay AA groups and "clean and sober" social events organized by lesbian communities seemed to absorb some of the social functions previously provided by the lesbian bar subculture. Lesbian-and-gay-only treatment programs, lesbian support groups, and various self-help or mutual-help groups were used by lesbians in recovery to make new friends and to stay in touch with lesbian community life in recovery. For some the social transition was a great upheaval and change, whereas for others it was a smooth move from a niche in one social milieu (the bar) to a similar role in the recovering lesbian community.

At first I was really interested in meeting lesbians in the AA groups. I was chasing the girls in the program, just like before.

For 9 years I hung out at the same lesbian bar on a daily basis. I would get there about 5 pm and sit talking to the owner until it got busy. There were about five of us regulars who did that. The owner was more than just an owner. She kept the community safe, and made sure we had this place where we could be ourselves. I couldn't imagine not going there every day. . . . When I quit drinking I found out there was this coffee shop where all the AA dykes hung out, and I was back in my element. It was even easier to be there than in the bars, because people would talk to you more willingly. And I discovered I could even sometimes go to the bars with lesbians in recovery, and not drink alcohol.

Now it's easier for lesbians to be sober because it has become a strong cultural value here on the coast. . . . I remember being at a party 2 years ago when, out of 15 women, I was the only one drinking. . . . Lesbians don't go to bars anymore, they go to AA meetings.

Part of recovery for me was learning not to go in bars, closing the doors I still had left open that could lead back to alcohol and drug use. I had to call my dealer up and say I wouldn't ever be talking to him again.

IMPLICATIONS FOR HEALTH CARE

Given the diversity of images for recovery that are relevant to lesbians who have alcohol problems, health care providers need to expand their awareness of recovery images and learn to apply these images more flexibly and interchangeably in their interactions with clients. Clients' images of recovery can be expected to change over time and circumstances, and individuals may hold several images simultaneously. These images are important ways in which change and stability are framed within personal and collective recovery experience. The provider who has a fixed theory or vision of what recovery is or should be unduly constrains the creative dimensions of the process in favor of a "recipe" approach. This is especially unsuitable for those whose life experiences differ significantly from the mainstream culture. Lesbians definitely fall into this category.

The uncritical promotion of AA and other Twelve Step groups as the single or even the best model of recovery is inappropriate. The Twelve Step model does not incorporate many of the images of recovery reflected by the lesbians whose experiences are described here. Recovery as vocational change, as empowerment, and as reclamation of the self or past are at best only partially or indirectly addressed by the Twelve Steps.

The conversion aspects of the AA view of recovery may falsely characterize past trauma experienced by these women, such as incest or other sexual abuse, as moral weakness or "character defects." Valuable survival strategies that were employed in the period of alcohol and drug use may unfortunately be rejected as remnants of the old self under the conversion image of recovery. Lesbians necessarily develop survival strategies to counter the damaging effects of social stigmatization. To think of beginning recovery as a new person, largely abandoning past ways of life, may not only present too great a threat to lesbians, but may inappropriately discount the validity of their experiences and the usefulness of their prior survival tactics. Although much of the stigma of having an alcohol problem abates when one begins recovery and finds a support group of other recovering persons, the stigma against being lesbian still operates in society, in health care contexts, and within Twelve Step groups as well.

Counseling, psychotherapy, social work, and nursing have offered important opportunities for lesbians to talk about recovery issues that are not easily addressed in the AA scenario. It is important that in becoming well versed about substance abuse issues these providers avoid packaging their wares exclusively in the language and principles of Twelve Step programs. If anything, more, not fewer, images of recovery are needed to validate the range of life experiences lesbians have had in this area. Those lesbians who have experienced a number of compulsive tendencies appreciate therapy that helps them make decisions that take all of their problems into consideration, without minimizing any, in a way that integrates strategies rather than fragments them.

For incest and other abuse survivors, interaction with providers not only offers an avenue for understanding some of the reasons why alcohol and drug use began and accelerated, but deals with the trauma in the larger sphere of life as a whole. There are legitimate times in recovery when the focus ought to be shifted away from the issues of drinking and drug use per se to more pervasive, lifelong difficulties that may have been engendered much earlier, in childhood. This does not necessarily mean that clients do not need to continue their recovery strategies for alcohol problems. Many lesbians report that during their work on incest, child abuse, etc., they experienced significant discomfort and anxiety but did not seriously consider substance use as an option. Provider fears that arousing these sleeping dogs will precipitate a substance abuse relapse do not appear to be well founded on the basis of these interviews. Just as images of recovery change and are expanded at various intervals for each individual, the emergence of earlier trauma issues seems to have its own natural timetable that sensitive providers wisely respect. In other words, the optimal time for past trauma issues to be addressed seems to be when the client begins to speak about them.

The notion of recovery as empowerment has not been effectively incorporated into most mainstream recovery programs. There are a few remarkable projects serving women and, in some cases, specifically lesbian clients (Sandmaier, 1980). They serve as models for how empowerment can be incorporated through group work and emphasis on feminist, antiracist principles. To be open and supportive of this image of recovery, providers must acknowledge that women are the best authorities regarding their own healing and liberation, a tenet that conflicts with the compliance and control so often used in clinical interaction. Health care providers must be open and responsive to critiques from clients regarding the racist, classist, and sexist aspects of treatment programs, Twelve Step programs, and policies affecting minority communities with regard to alcohol and other drug use.

Recovery as social transition is uniquely expressed among lesbians, because it reflects the cultural developmental processes that are currently creating drug- and alcohol-free social structures in lesbian communities. The closure of many lesbian bars, the institution of clean and sober lesbian social environments, and the influence of lesbians on the organization and practices of Twelve Step programs are aspects of social transition at the collective level. Individually, lesbians must negotiate the transition from drinking to recovery in the face of social obstacles such as economic pressure, lack of lesbian-sensitive treatment programs, prejudices of health care providers, the white male biases of some AA members, and, for some, even the tension of seeing their self-conflicts reflected in lesbian AA meetings.

Lesbians in recovery also have some unique images of recovery involving celebration. The impact of Living Sober, with its openness to address the interests of so many subgroups of lesbians and gay men within Twelve Step programs, including the development of theater and artwork as expressions of recovery, is in fact influencing and reshaping AA as a whole. Albeit slowly, lesbians and gay men are challenging AA's straight, white, male Christian assumptions by publicly celebrating the existence of minorities within AA.

At the community level, outreach, education, and prevention efforts concerning alcohol problems must also expand images of recovery. The fragmentation of programs, each addressing a specific compulsive problem, may be unnecessarily expensive and ineffective. Exclusive dependence on Twelve Step programs as the foundation of other interventions may alienate minority groups who want recovery but do not wish to use the Twelve Step programs. Lesbian communities represent an excellent example of community-based efforts to face alcohol problems. They have organized themselves to combat a problem they perceive as a personal, social, and political threat to their health. If more resources could be made available to lesbian communities, it is certain that many creative new interventions for outreach, treatment, mutual support, and social alternatives to drinking and drug use would be developed by these communities themselves.

REFERENCES

Alcoholics Anonymous World Services. (1976). *Alcoholics Anonymous* (3rd Ed.). New York: Author.

Bradford, J., & Ryan, C. (1988). *The national lesbian health care survey.* Washington, DC: National Lesbian and Gay Health Foundation.

Burke, P. (1982, April). *Bar use and alienation in lesbians and heterosexual women alcoholics.* Paper presented at the 30th National Alcohol Forum, Washington, DC.

Cantu, C. (1985). *Substance abuse issues among women: A brief overview* (Community Substance Abuse Services report). San Francisco: Division of Alcohol Programs.

Earle, R. M. (1982). Prevention of alcoholism in the United States and the National Council on Alcoholism: 1944–1950. *International Journal of the Addictions, 17,* 679–702.

Fifield, L. H., Latham, J. D., & Phillips, C. (1977). *Alcoholism and the gay community: The price of alienation, isolation, and oppression* (California Department of Alcohol and Drug Problems contract 76-56643). Los Angeles: Gay Community Services Center.

Hall, J. M. (1990a). Alcoholism in lesbians: Developmental, symbolic interactionist, and critical perspectives. *Health Care for Women International, 11,* 89–107.

Hall, J. M. (1990b). Alcoholism recovery in lesbian women: A theory in development. *Scholarly Inquiry for Nursing Practice: An International Journal, 4*(2), 109–125.

Hall, J. M. (1991). *Lesbians and alcohol: Patterns and paradoxes in medical notions and lesbian beliefs.* Manuscript submitted for publication.

Hastings, P. (1982, August 18). Alcohol and the lesbian community: Changing patterns of awareness. *Drinking and Drug Practices Surveyor,* pp. 3–7.

Hepburn, C., & Gutierrez, B. (1988). *Alive and well: A lesbian health guide.* Freedom, CA: Crossing Press.

Herman, E. (1988). Getting to serenity: Do addiction programs sap our political vitality? *Outlook: National Gay and Lesbian Quarterly, 1*(2), 10–21.

James, W. (1961). *The varieties of religious experience: A study in human nature.* New York: Collier Books. (Original work published 1902.)

Jellinek, E. M. (1960). *The disease concept of alcoholism.* New Haven, CT: College & University Press.

Johnson, S. R., & Palermo, J. L. (1984). Gynecologic care for the lesbian. *Clinical Obstetrics and Gynecology, 27,* 724–731.

Kurtz, E. (1988). *A.A. The story: A revised edition of "Not-God: A history of Alcoholics Anonymous."* San Francisco: Harper & Row.

Levine, H. G. (1984). The alcohol problem in America: From temperance to alcoholism. *British Journal of Addiction, 79,* 109–119.

Maxwell, M. A. (1984). *The Alcoholics Anonymous experience: A close-up view for professionals.* New York: McGraw-Hill.

McKirnan, D. J., & Peterson, P. L. (1989a). Alcohol and drug use among homosexual men and women: Epidemiology and population characteristics. *Addictive Behaviors, 14,* 545–553.

McKirnan, D. J., & Peterson, P. L. (1989b). Psychosocial and social factors in alcohol and drug abuse: An analysis of a homosexual community. *Addictive Behaviors, 14,* 555–563.

McNally, E. B. (1989). *Lesbian recovering alcoholics in Alcoholics Anonymous: A qualitative study of identity transformation.* Unpublished doctoral dissertation. School of Education, Health, Nursing, and Arts Professions, New York University, New York.

Morales, E. S., & Graves, M. A. (1983). *Substance abuse: Patterns and barriers to treatment for gay men and lesbians.* San Francisco: Department of Public Health, Community Substance Abuse Services.

Morin, S. F. (1977). Heterosexual bias in psychological research on lesbian and male homosexuality. *American Psychologist, 32,* 629–637.

Nardi, P. M. (1982). Alcoholism and homosexuality: A theoretical perspective. *Journal of Homosexuality, 7*(4), 9–26.

Nicoloff, L. K., & Stiglitz, E. A. (1987). Lesbian alcoholism: Etiology, treatment, and recovery. In Boston Lesbian Psychologies Collective (Eds.), *Lesbian psychologies* (pp. 283–293). Urbana, IL: University of Illinois Press.

Peele, S. (1986). The implications and limitations of genetic models of alcoholism and other addictions. *Journal of Studies on Alcohol, 47*(1), 63–73.

Room, R. (1988, September). *Cultural changes in drinking and trends in alcohol prob-lems indicators: Recent U.S. experience.* Paper presented at an International Work-shop of Alcohol Epidemiological Studies, Greve-in-Chianti, Italy.

Royce, J. E. (1986). Sin or solace: Religious views on alcohol and alcoholism. In T. D. Watts (Ed.), *Social thought on alcoholism: A comprehensive review* (pp. 53–66). Malabar, FL: Robert E. Krieger.

Rudy, D. (1986). *Becoming alcoholic: Alcoholics Anonymous and the reality of alcohol-ism.* Carbondale, IL: Southern Illinois University Press.

Saghir, M. T., & Robins, E. (1973). *Male and female homosexuality: A comprehensive investigation.* Baltimore, MD: Williams & Wilkins.

Sandmaier, M. (1980). *The invisible alcoholics: Women and alcohol abuse in America.* New York: McGraw-Hill.

Schilit, R., Clark, W. M., & Shallenberger, E. A. (1988). Social supports and lesbian alcoholics. *Affilia, 3*(2), 27–40.

Shaffer, H. J. (1986). Conceptual crises and the addictions: A philosophy of science perspective. *Journal of Substance Abuse Treatment, 3,* 285–296.

Stevens, P. E., & Hall, J. M. (1988). Stigma, health beliefs, and experiences with health care in lesbian women. *Image: Journal of Nursing Scholarship, 20*(2), 69–73.

Stevens, P. E., & Hall, J. M. (1991). A critical historical analysis of the medical construction of lesbianism. *International Journal of Health Services, 21,* 291–307.

Szasz, T. (1970). *The manufacture of madness: A comparative study of the Inquisition and the mental health movement.* New York: Delta.

Thune, C. E. (1977). Alcoholism and the archetypal past: A phenomenological perspec-tive on Alcoholics Anonymous. *Journal of Studies on Alcohol, 38*(1), 75–88.

Tomko, M. K. (1988). Recovery: A multidimensional process. *Issues in Mental Health Nursing, 9*(2), 139–149.

Vourakis, C. (1989). *Process of recovery for women in AA: Seeking groups "like me."* Unpublished doctoral dissertation, School of Nursing, University of California, San Francisco.

Weathers, B. (1976). *Alcoholism and the lesbian community: Needs report.* Los Angeles: Alcoholism Center for Women.

Wilson-Schaef, A. (1987). *When society becomes an addict.* San Francisco: Harper & Row.

Ziebold, T. (1979, January). Alcoholism and recovery: Gays helping gays. *Christopher Street,* pp. 36–44.

HOW DO LESBIAN WOMEN DEVELOP SERENITY?

Sharon Deevey, RN, MS
College of Nursing, Ohio State University, Columbus, Ohio

Lana J. Wall, MSW
Alpatha Healing Center and Union Institute, Columbus, Ohio

This article considers how lesbian women recover from alcoholism and develop serenity in the context of a homophobic society. We review what is known about the incidence and lethality of alcoholism in lesbian women. We critique Finnegan and McNally's (1987) five-stage conceptual framework of lesbian and alcoholic identity development, which is based on the disease model of recovery. We present our own model, based on our own recovery experiences. The Deevey–Wall model describes factors that may determine how shaming social environments may affect drinking behavior and recovery in lesbian women. In conclusion, we explain Wall's theory of self-hate as a survival mechanism in traumatically hostile environments.

Lesbian women are recognized as an at-risk population in recent health care literature. After years of public silence and medical misinformation about the life reality of lesbian women, lesbian community advocates (O'Donnell, Leoffler, Pollock, & Saunders, 1979) and clinical researchers (Johnson, Smith, & Guenther, 1987) have brought the health concerns of lesbian women to the attention of professional caregivers. Homophobia, or negative attitudes and behaviors toward lesbian and gay people, is identified as (a) a major stress on the physical and mental health of lesbian women (Bradford & Ryan, 1988) and (b) the reason many lesbian women avoid contact with health care professionals (Kavanagh, 1979; Randall, 1989; Stevens & Hall, 1988).

Alcohol abuse is a primary health problem in lesbian communities. The earliest recognition of this problem emerged outside the medical mainstream in the pamphlets of the self-help and women's movements (Schwartz, 1980; Swallow, 1983). It is estimated that at least 30% of lesbian women may be considered alcoholic, and several authors have examined the relationship between alcohol abuse and familial, social, and emotional factors in lesbian women (Diamond & Wilsnack, 1987; Glaus, 1989; Haven, 1981; Israelstrom & Lambert, 1986; Kus, 1985; Woods, 1981).

Accurate statistics are difficult to obtain because of the hidden nature of the lesbian community, disagreement about definitions of alcohol use and abuse, and the great variety in age of recognition and acceptance of lesbian identity. Alcoholism in women in general has also been more hidden and more stigmatized than alcoholism in men.

Several reasons for the high incidence of alcoholism among lesbian women have been proposed in the anecdotal and research literature. For many years, urban bars were the only "safe" place for lesbian women to meet and be together outside private homes. Schwartz (1980) explained that "the gay bar is to many gay men and lesbian women what the country club, church picnic, or community center is to heterosexuals" (p. 4). Older lesbian women in particular had few alternatives to bars in their younger years. Schwartz also explained how denial of alcoholism may be greater in lesbian and gay individuals than in the general population: Because lesbian women become skilled at "denying that they are bothered by society's attitudes toward them, [this] makes it easier to deny that they are abusing alcohol" (p. 4).

Oppression is thought to contribute to alcoholism in lesbian women in two other ways. Drinking is used to cope with the stress, alienation, and despair of rejection by society. Nicoloff and Stiglitz (1987) argued, "On a political level, minority groups are forced into addiction. Drugs and alcohol are provided in order to keep people under control. . . . the job of the oppressor becomes easier when individuals engage in self-destructive behaviors and render themselves powerless" (p. 286).

Rofes (1983) and Saunders and Valente (1987) stated that alcohol abuse is frequently a contributing factor in lesbian and gay suicide, which is estimated to be two to seven times higher than in heterosexuals. The combination of high incidence and potentially high lethality make alcohol abuse a significant health problem for the population of lesbian women.

What helps lesbian women who have misused alcohol develop sobriety and serenity? How is the process of recovery affected by the interaction of alcoholism and lesbian issues? What other factors complicate or contribute to recovery in this population? Two models are presented in this article to provide caregivers some insight into these questions.

FINNEGAN–McNALLY MODEL

Finnegan and McNally (1987) proposed a five-stage conceptual model to help caregivers of lesbian and gay clients in treatment programs understand the interaction between the "misery of alcoholism" and the "grinding oppression of homophobia" (see Figure 1). Figure 1 represents our summary of the Finnegan–McNally model. In the first stage, "pre-encounter," the individual lacks self-awareness about either alcoholism or lesbian issues. She identifies with the values of the majority, often condemning "drunks" and "homosexuals," while assuming her "social drinker" and "heterosexual" identities. Stage 2, "encounter," is the shock of recognizing she is different from others, either in being unable to control her drinking or in becoming aware of lesbian sexual feelings. In Stage 3, "immersion/emersion," the individual is reactively militant about being different, condemning and avoiding "earth people" (nonalcoholics) and the "straight" (nonlesbian) world. In Stage 4, "internalization," the individual grieves for the loss of normalcy and the other losses that accompany stigma. Stage 5, "synthesis/ commitment," is the acceptance of being different; being alcoholic and lesbian is peacefully and often openly acknowledged. In this last stage,

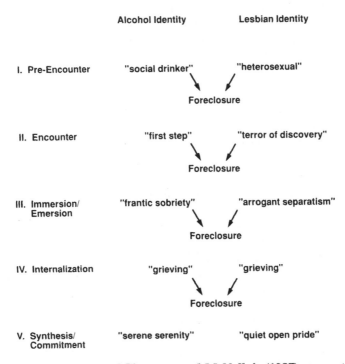

Figure 1. A summary of Finnegan and McNally's (1987) conceptualization of alcohol identity development and lesbian identity development in recovering alcoholic lesbian women.

the rest of the world is no longer seen as "similar to me" or "different from me," but instead is accurately assessed as supportive or nonsupportive.

Although presented for simplicity as a linear model, Finnegan and McNally (1987) explained that their model describes stages that are "not distinct entities"; movement within the stages can be "fluid." An individual usually does not go through the stages of alcohol and lesbian identity development simultaneously. Many arrogantly separatist lesbian militants (L3) are heavy drinkers with no knowledge of addiction recovery (A1). Many women have 2 to 3 years of somewhat frantic sobriety (A3) or "unexplained" relapses before they tentatively enter the encounter stage of first acknowledging their lesbian identity (L1).

Finnegan and McNally (1987) also explained that not all lesbian or gay people go through all the stages: "[Some] stay in one stage all their lives, and some do just fine in that stage" (p. 79). Others "foreclose," which is defined as blocking further knowledge or growth by denial, continued substance abuse, medical or religious redefinition, or the pretense of heterosexuality. In many parts of the United States, foreclosure in the encounter (L2, "terror of discovery") stage is the norm for most lesbian women. Open acceptance of lesbian identity is not considered an option or goal; in fact, openly lesbian women are sometimes shunned by closeted lesbian women (McDaniel, 1985).

Finnegan and McNally (1987) suggested that when lesbian and gay people do foreclose,

> the power of denial is tremendous. People have . . . an enormous investment in being okay in the eyes of the world and themselves. Their psychic survival depends on denial and any other defense which helps them block the terrifying knowledge of who they are or might be. (p. 80)

Finnegan and McNally suggested that the insensitive caregiver who prematurely confronts sexual identity issues can push "an already frightened and vulnerable person over the brink and into the pit of homophobic shame" (p. 81).

We have used the Finnegan–McNally (1987) model to make sense of our own experience as lesbian women recovering from alcohol abuse. It is our contention, however, that although this model is a pioneering contribution, it fails to offer sufficient explanation of the problem of alcohol abuse in lesbian communities. This model seems to accept the disease model of alcoholism, despite the clear awareness of the interaction of how lesbian identity development complicates recovery from substance abuse. We believe that it is inaccurate to conclude that 30% of lesbian women develop the "disease" of alcoholism while disregarding the social context in which lesbian women drink. The disease model, including Finnegan and McNally's version, describes alcoholism as an individual process of illness and recovery. This perspective has been useful in recovery, but ignores some important questions about the impact of varying environments on individuals. The disease model also focuses only on those most severely disabled by alcohol abuse and ignores the many individuals whose emotional growth is retarded by the use of alcohol as a primary method of coping with prejudice.

The Finnegan–McNally (1987) model fails to answer the broader questions about how a shaming social environment affects drinking behaviors in individuals who are despised by the majority. Current homophobic cultural values generate a constant barrage of shaming messages that label the lesbian (or gay) individual as perverted, disgusting, sinful, criminal, diseased, dangerous, unpatriotic, or nonexistent. In such an environment it is no surprise that shame, or internalized homophobia, leads to foreclosure and blocks self-acceptance in lesbian and gay people.

To understand the big picture of alcohol abuse in lesbian women, several additional questions need to be asked: What societal factors contribute to foreclosure? What combination of individual and community factors influence the acceptance or rejection of shaming homophobic messages? Is there a difference in family background, coping skills, or educational level between lesbian women who reach serenity and open pride and those who drink heavily or remain deeply closeted? Do geography and the varying levels of homophobia in different communities really make a difference? How does alcohol interact with these individual, family, and community factors? How can caregivers predict which individuals will progress, and which will self-destruct? Finally, are there individual or environmental interventions to help lesbian women reach serenity?

DEEVEY–WALL MODEL

The Deevey–Wall model (see Figure 2) represents our initial effort to grapple with these questions. In this model, the young individual receives constant shaming messages from society. Acceptance or rejection of the shaming messages is mediated by factors that are both internal and external to the individual. Internal factors may include physical status, personality, family history, education, or coping skills. For example, socially valued physical assets like beauty, strength, or wellness may support rejection of homophobic messages, whereas physical disability or illness may increase vulnerability to shame. Personality may also affect the acceptance or rejection of shaming messages; for example, lesbian extroverts who are often less comfortable in the closet than

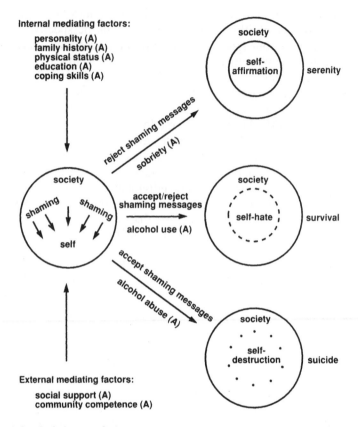

Figure 2. The Deevey–Wall model: internal, external, and alcohol factors in the development of serenity in lesbian women.

the quieter introverts may be more motivated to work toward openness on sexual orientation issues.

Family history and education may be important factors in how one deals in general with communication, conflict, and change. Individuals raised in families with open communication, negotiated conflict, and positive attitudes toward change may be less vulnerable to shame. Knowledge about the existence and history of sexual minorities determines how abnormal or ordinary one initially feels as a lesbian or gay person. An individual with greater learning skills may be more able to locate validating written information about lesbian and gay history. A wide variety of coping skills may help an individual deflect shaming messages with humor, diversionary activity, or confrontation. Knowledge about emotions and practice expressing them directly may also be determined by education and coping skills and may then influence acceptance or rejection of shaming messages.

External mediating factors include social support and community competence. Social support includes the people (and their emotional and financial resources) who are available to the lesbian or gay person. Family of origin, friends, work colleagues, and children may support the lesbian or gay person in rejecting shaming messages or, of course, may be the source of them. Community competence is how well a community protects its diverse members, in this case from abuse by homophobic individuals and institutions. Community competence includes religious and legal support for lesbian rights, the existence of knowledgeable public and private health care agencies, sufficient economic resources, and the ability of the community to respond to violence and disease. Communities vary enormously in the information and resources available for lesbian women and thereby influence the "choice" an individual has about foreclosure or self-acceptance.

Alcohol may be a cofactor in both internal and external factors. We believe that sobriety is essential in the development of serenity; at present, at least, we know of no lesbian women who use alcohol who seem fully self-accepting. We see alcohol use as one of several strategies for coping with the self-hate of simultaneously accepting and rejecting shaming messages. Alcohol use in combination with accepting shaming messages leads either to active suicide or to indirect suicide as a result of the progression of alcoholism. Alcohol may also be a cofactor in physical status (genetic sensitivity), family history (alcoholic parents or grandparents), and education (information about addiction learned in school). Alcohol may be a cofactor in social support (familial or collegial support for either alcohol use or sobriety) and community competence (treatment programs and community knowledge).

Research is needed to determine whether our model is useful in explaining or predicting who among lesbian women will reach sobriety, self-acceptance, and serenity. In the meantime, intervention will continue to be merely hopeful and haphazard until more is understood about the process. In our experience, one intriguing aspect of the model that needs further consideration is the role of self-hate in the development of serenity. Managing the conflict of both accepting and rejecting shaming messages leads to self-hate. Although self-hate blocks self-affirmation, it also prevents self-destruction and therefore, paradoxically, is crucial for survival.

Wall (1986) offered an explanation for how self-hate functions as a similar survival mechanism in childhood incest survivors. Wall argued that the child experiencing incest is completely powerless to control her situation, except by blaming (and therefore hating) herself. Self-blame (self-hate) allows the child to perceive control through the explanation that she is responsible; otherwise, the experience is so traumatizing that the child cannot survive. The child cannot blame the parent/perpetrator because, in reality, the child cannot survive independently. Self-hate therefore gives the child the perception of control and becomes a detriment only later in life. The insensitive caregiver who pushes the incest survivor to give up self-hate without recognizing its adaptive function may force the client into suicidal crisis. The sensitive caregiver will teach the incest survivor about the survival mechanism of self-hate and support the client's growth toward other ways of coping with both the remembered reality of childhood powerlessness and the current challenges of adult living.

There are clear parallels between Wall's explanation of self-hate in incest survivors and self-hate in lesbian women. Many lesbian individuals are adolescents or adults before their first recognition of their sexual orientation. In many ways, however, the newly self-aware lesbian perceives she is as alone and powerless in the midst of heterosexual society as is the child in a dysfunctional family. Survival for the lesbian woman depends on living and working in a society that is traumatically hostile to the lesbian or gay person. Because she cannot survive outside society, the lesbian woman blames (and therefore hates) herself in order to perceive control in an otherwise intolerable situation.

The sensitive caregiver needs to teach lesbian women how self-hate serves, at least initially, as a survival mechanism. Lesbian women also need to be warned of the dangers of using alcohol as a primary way of coping with prejudice and need to be taught how internal and external mediating factors like those in the model may block or promote emotional growth. Lesbian women who have achieved sobriety and self-affirmation need to be visible, to be role models of a self-acceptance unimaginable to lesbian women in the first stages of coming out. Lesbian women must recognize the ways in which society is dysfunctional, much as incest survivors must confront the dysfunction in their families.

Lesbian women experience a long and arduous journey through hostile territory, from the pit of homophobic shame to self-affirmation and serenity. Like any life-threatening journey, the process can be a complex mixture of menace and exhilaration. Although many foreclose, and some die by their own hand along the way, others survive, and more and more are reaching a self-affirming serenity.

Those of us who have reached a certain serenity look back with wonder and gratitude for our escape from self-hate; we remember with anguish those lesbian loved ones who died or who are self-destructing in their journey. We hope, in this article, to offer an initial roadmap to help lesbian women and their caregivers negotiate the uncharted territory from the first solitary experience of lesbian shaming to the serenity of lesbian self-affirmation, one day at a time.

REFERENCES

Bradford, J., & Ryan, C. (1988). *The national lesbian health care survey.* Washington, DC: National Lesbian and Gay Health Foundation.

Diamond, D. L., & Wilsnack, S. C. (1987). Alcohol use among lesbians: A descriptive study. *Journal of Homosexuality, 4*(2), 123–142.

Finnegan, D. G., & McNally, E. B. (1987). *Dual identities: Counseling chemically dependent gay men and lesbians.* Center City, MN: Hazelden.

Glaus, K. O. (1989). Alcoholism, chemical dependency, and the lesbian client. *Women and Therapy, 8*(1–2), 131–144.

Haven, M. J. (1981). Alcoholism and self-esteem among women with a female sex object preference. *Dissertation Abstracts International, 42,* 2058B.

Israelstrom, S., & Lambert, S. (1986). Homosexuality and alcohol: Observations and research after the psychoanalytic era. *International Journal of the Addictions, 21,* 509–537.

Johnson, S. R., Smith, E. M., & Guenther, S. M. (1987). Comparison of gynecologic health care problems between lesbians and bisexual women: A survey of 2,345 women. *Journal of Reproductive Medicine, 32,* 805–811.

Kavanagh, J. (1979). *Lesbians' attitudes and experiences concerning traditional health care.* Unpublished master's thesis, Case Western Reserve University, Cleveland, OH.

Kus, R. J. (1985). Stages of coming out: An ethnographic approach. *Western Journal of Nursing Research, 7,* 177–198.

McDaniel, J. (1985). My life as the only lesbian professor. In M. Cruikshank (Ed.), *The lesbian path* (pp. 160–165). San Francisco, CA: Grey Fox Press.

Nicoloff, L. K., & Stiglitz, E. A. (1987). Lesbian alcoholism: Etiology, treatment, and recovery. In Boston Lesbian Psychologies Collective (Ed.), *Lesbian psychologies* (pp. 283–293). Urbana, IL: University of Illinois Press.

O'Donnell, M., Loeffler, V., Pollock, K., & Saunders, Z. (1979). *Lesbian health matters!* Santa Cruz, CA: Santa Cruz Women's Health Collective.

Randall, C. E. (1989). Lesbianphobia among BSN educators: A survey. *Journal of Nursing Education, 28,* 302–306.

Rofes, E. E. (1983). *I thought people like that killed themselves: Lesbians, gay men, and suicide.* San Francisco, CA: Grey Fox Press.

Saunders, J. M., & Valente, S. M. (1987). Suicide risk among gay men and lesbians: A review. *Death Studies, 11,* 1–23.

Schwartz, L. R. (1980). *Alcoholism among lesbians/gay men: A critical problem in critical proportions.* Phoenix, AZ: Do It Now Foundation.

Stevens, P. E., & Hall, J. M. (1988). Stigma, health beliefs, and experiences with health care in lesbian women. *Image: Journal of Nursing Scholarship, 20*(2), 69–73.

Swallow, J. (Ed.). (1983). *Out from under: Sober dykes and our friends.* San Francisco: Spinsters/Aunt Lute.

Wall, L. J. (1986, June). *Victimization and survival.* Workshop presented at Ohio Drug and Alcohol Studies Institute, Kenyon College, Gambier, OH.

Woods, C. P. (1981). Alcohol use among lesbians: An investigation of contributing factors. *Dissertation Abstracts International, 42,* 2558B.

LESBIAN CHILDBEARING COUPLES'
DILEMMAS AND DECISIONS

Janet W. Kenney, RN, PhD, and Donna T. Tash, RN, CNM

College of Nursing, Arizona State University, Tempe, Arizona

In recent years, an increasing number of lesbian women have chosen to bear children. However, for lesbians, there are many obstacles and unique dilemmas during each phase of the childbearing process. Some of these dilemmas include how to conceive, where to find a health care provider who is sensitive to their concerns, and how to inform family members and friends about the pregnancy and elicit their support. Other dilemmas common to all women are where to give birth and how to assimilate new roles into their life and work. This article describes the potential dilemmas of lesbians during childbearing, with the aim of increasing health care providers' awareness of and sensitivity to the perinatal concerns of lesbian women.

It has been estimated that 2–12% of all American women are lesbians and that about one third of all lesbians are mothers (Hall, 1978). A recent survey of 2,000 lesbians and bisexuals stated that a majority of these women desire to have children (Johnson, Smith, & Guenther, 1987). The number of lesbian couples choosing to bear children has increased. These couples face numerous health care dilemmas during each phase of the childbearing process. Some dilemmas unique to lesbian women are how to conceive, where to find a lesbian-sensitive health care provider, and how to handle their personal, family, and lesbian social relationships. Other dilemmas common to all women include where to give birth and how to assimilate new roles and responsibilities into their life and employment.

There are only a few published studies of lesbians' unique gynecological and obstetrical health care needs. Most of these studies included predominantly white, middle-class lesbians, between the ages of 20 and 45, who were college-educated professionals (Harvey, Carr, & Bernheime, 1989; Olesker & Walsh, 1984; Smith, Johnson, & Guenther, 1985; Trippet & Bain, 1990). Although these studies usually were based on small, self-selected samples, some common themes and psychosocial health concerns of lesbians were identified. For example, many lesbians reported fear that their health care would be jeopardized if they revealed their sexual orientation to their provider. In addition, they felt providers lacked practical knowledge about lesbians and were insensitive to their health concerns (Harvey et al., 1989; Smith et al., 1985). Because of the paucity of information about the dilemmas and needs of childbearing lesbians, along with blatant discrimination and prejudiced attitudes, lesbian childbearing couples are at risk for receiving less than optimal health care.

Our purpose in this article is to provide a cogent summary of the literature on lesbian childbearing couples, integrating practice-based knowledge of pregnant lesbian couples. The major dilemmas and decisions lesbian childbearing couples may face are presented in the four sequential phases of childbearing. In the first phase, lesbian couples must make an active decision to become parents and explore their options for achieving conception. During pregnancy, both heterosexual and lesbian couples explore their desires for an idealized pregnancy and delivery experience. However, lesbian couples try to find a health care provider who will affirm their values and relationship. Also, they may decide to assimilate into traditional childbirth classes. Both heterosexual and lesbian couples must decide whether to deliver at home, in a birthing center, or in a hospital; however, lesbians fear ostracism and mistreatment by traditional health care providers. Last, dilemmas may arise after the birth, including concerns over coparenting, adoption by one's partner, and acceptance by one's family of origin and by the lesbian community.

LESBIAN'S VIEWS OF HEALTH
AND HEALTH CARE PROVIDERS

The majority of lesbian health care studies have sampled white, well-educated, middle-class women; therefore, the health care views reflect the attitudes of this population. In a study of 25 midwestern lesbians, health was conceptualized in a holistic fashion, with an emphasis on independence and self-reliance (Stevens & Hall, 1988). Athleticism, physical exercise, and good nutrition were viewed as physical health strengths.

Several studies have shown that lesbians prefer alternative health care practices such as homeopathy, chiropractic, and midwifery (Olesker & Walsh, 1984; Smith et al., 1985; Stevens & Hall, 1988). Lesbians prefer lesbian gynecologists and midwives, who affirm their health values and support their life-style. They often choose nontraditional health care services to avoid adverse interaction with the physician/provider (Harvey et al., 1989). One study of 43 lesbians reported that 37% did not have a regular health care provider because of the high cost and lack of need for services (Trippet & Bain, 1990). Lesbians may avoid the mainstream patriarchal health services because of an overwhelming mistrust of its ability to provide safe and adequate care for them if their sexual orientation becomes known. Many lesbians fear disclosure of their sexual orientation and conceal their life-style when they sense discomfort or subtle signs of disapproval. Also, they may fear that their health problem will be interpreted as a pathological extension of their lesbian life-style (Stevens & Hall, 1988).

Two studies reported that 40–72% of lesbians surveyed received negative responses from health care providers after revealing their sexual orientation (Smith et al., 1985; Stevens & Hall, 1988). In Stevens and Hall's (1988) study, lesbians described ostracism, invasive personal questions, shock, embarrassment, unfriendliness, pity, condescension, and fear from health care providers. Lesbians also reported that their partners had been mistreated, their confidentiality had been breached, and they had experienced rough physical handling and derogatory comments. After a lifetime of negative, derogatory responses from health care providers and society, lesbians have developed a sensitivity to these potential risks and thus seek ways to minimize their exposure to them. In choosing to conceive and bear children, lesbians increase their risk of exposure to and ostracism by health care providers.

CONCEPTION: DILEMMAS AND DECISIONS

Several studies have reported that many lesbians not only have a desire to parent, but also want to experience pregnancy and childbirth (Harvey et al., 1989; Olesker & Walsh, 1984). Some reasons that lesbians gave for choosing to parent biologically include their concerns about early infant bonding, the lack of adoption alternatives, and the desire to raise a newborn (Harvey et al., 1989). Reasons given for their decision to become parents include the love of children, belief in their ability to be good parents, a desire to pass on their own values, and the desire for stability in their lives (Olesker & Walsh, 1984).

Whereas some lesbians have had children from former heterosexual marriages, other lesbians have never had any children; their desire to experience pregnancy and/or parenting may be great. Among lesbians, achieving conception requires much forethought and planning. Lesbian couples must weigh their desire to coparent and consider the effects of children on their relationship, life-style, and network of friends. Some lesbian couples decide not to become parents because they fear their own parents' reactions (or anticipated reactions).

After choosing to become pregnant, the lesbian couple must then decide whether to use artificial insemination or sexual intercourse. If the couple decides on artificial insemination, as the majority of women in Harvey et al.'s (1989) study did, they may have to use the traditional patriarchal health care system. Because the present health care system is defined and administered by mostly middle- to upper-class, traditional, heterosexual, white males, most lesbians expect to encounter barriers to insemination services. According to Zook and Hallenback (1987), lesbian couples reported difficulty finding health care providers who would support their concept of family. Health care systems may deny access, lack sensitivity, and communicate disrespect. Many clinics refuse to offer insemination services to all unmarried women, including lesbians.

The cost of artificial insemination is another concern for lesbians. Some women are unable to take advantage of group insurance and may have difficulty obtaining care at a fee that is affordable to them. Also, very few insurance companies pay for sperm, which is the major expense.

In choosing artificial insemination, lesbians must decide whether to use a known or unknown donor. In the Harvey et al. (1989) study, 83% of the women conceived through artificial insemination; of these, 66% used an unknown donor. Other studies reported 11% (Olesker & Walsh, 1984) and 41% (Johnson et al., 1987) of lesbian couples used artificial insemination. Some lesbians choose to use the semen from a known male donor and inseminate with a turkey baster to avoid the medical expense of insemination. Lesbians reported that they chose donor insemination because they were reluctant or unwilling to engage in sexual intercourse (Harvey et al., 1989). Reasons for insemination with an unknown donor include the desire for confidentiality or avoiding potential coparenting complications. Recently, some lesbian couples have questioned the practice of using semen donated by homosexual men because of the potential for transmission of acquired immune deficiency syndrome (AIDS) from this high-risk group (Loulan, 1987). Use of frozen sperm, which is tested 6 months later, may reduce the risk of AIDS transmission. However, when unknown donors are used for insemination, children may grow up wondering about one half of their genetic background.

Conception by coitus was used by 8 of the 9 women in Olesker and Walsh's (1984) study. Males were chosen after exploring their health status, family history, intelligence, and personality. Although most of these women did not want male involvement, their reasons for using coitus were fear of unknown history of donor, fear of refusal to inseminate by health care provider, and difficulty arranging transport and insemination by someone other than a physician. In 7 of the 8 cases, the male was not aware of the desire for pregnancy, yet all but one male was informed afterward. These women did not expect financial remuneration or responsibility from the male.

If coitus or known donor insemination is used, lesbian couples have several realistic fears. For example, they may worry about future loss of custody to the semen donor or paternal involvement (Pollack, 1987), although some lesbians have encouraged continued relationships of the father with the child (Van Gelder, 1991). Also, the nonbiological lesbian parent may feel less important to the child, and the child may feel rejected by an uninvolved father if the biological father is known.

In choosing pregnancy, a lesbian couple may hope to acquire acceptance of the pregnancy by their own family of origin, a health care provider, and the gay community. According to Wismont and Reame (1989), "There may be disengagement by the couple from those within their social group who are not supportive of their parenting decision" (p. 138). Opposition from friends may be based on concerns over the couple's personal motivation, the child's sex role development, or fears of reduced political activism (Murphy, 1987; Pollack, 1987). Also, the gay community may feel the lesbian couple will favor friendships with heterosexual mothers, thus weakening the solidarity of their association with the gay community (Hill, 1987; Pollack, 1987). Loss of support by the lesbian community is very difficult to replace.

PREGNANCY: DILEMMAS AND DECISIONS

Once conception is achieved, the lesbian couple may consider whether they want delivery to occur in their home, a birthing center, or a hospital. Finding an accessible health provider who values and supports lesbian parenting, is sensitive to their unique needs, and is willing to attend the birth in the desired setting is often a difficult task. In a study of 36 childbearing lesbians, Harvey et al. (1989) reported that 52% sought care from physicians, and 48% chose nurse-midwives or lay-midwives. Initially, 11% of these lesbians were refused prenatal care by health care practitioners. All but 1 of 9 lesbians in Olesker and Walsh's (1984) study chose midwives for their care and reported high levels of support from and satisfaction with the midwives. Because many lesbian couples desire a home birth or birthing room experience, with minimal technological intervention, they are more likely than heterosexual women to choose midwives for their obstetrical care.

Once pregnancy was achieved, prenatal care was sought in the first trimester by almost 100% of the lesbians in two studies (Harvey et al.,

1989; Olesker & Walsh, 1984). Lesbians appear to be aware of the importance of and to be motivated to obtain health care early in their pregnancies. They place a high value on their own health and want a healthy infant. These couples sought health care providers who would encourage their active involvement during the pregnancy. However, they were concerned that if they did not reveal their sexual orientation, providers would assume they were heterosexual and direct their care toward that assumption (Olesker & Walsh, 1984). Another annoying problem lesbians encountered in traditional health care systems was exclusion of their female partner during examinations and counseling.

Childbirth education classes were attended by 89–100% of lesbians in two studies (Harvey et al., 1989; Olesker & Walsh, 1984). This would be expected of a group that places a high value on health and education. However, these classes tend to attract and be geared toward heterosexual couples, and none of the lesbian couples felt comfortable sharing their sexual orientation. Because they did not reveal their true relationship in these classes, they were perceived and accepted as single mothers. This may have created some discomfort along with denial of self.

Adjustment to the physical and psychological changes during pregnancy may require lesbian couples to adapt or modify their roles and relationship. During pregnancy, some women turn inward and focus on changes in their body functions and image, while others radiate outward and bask in their feelings of joy. Those who turn inward may expect unconditional emotional support and nurturance from their partners, including acceptance of their accompanying physical changes. Empathic partners may assimilate the emotional changes and experiences of the pregnant mother. However, some partners may feel rejected by their pregnant partner's self-centeredness, especially if diminished sexual desires accompany these changes. For other couples, where the pregnancy is strongly desired by both partners, it has been suggested that lesbian women have a better understanding of pregnancy and can provide more nurturing and cuddling than heterosexual men (Tolor & Degrazia, 1976).

What is different for pregnancy in lesbian couples is the lack of acknowledgment of the parental role of the nonbiological parent, especially in their work situation. Also, the lesbian couple may not have support from their families of origin and may feel anxious about telling their own parents that they will soon be grandparents.

As with heterosexual couples, jealousy of the pregnancy or future infant, along with fear of diminished love or abandonment, may interfere with the lesbian couple's relationship. Although the couple may have mutually decided on the pregnancy, they cannot always predict their reactions to the changing circumstances. Sometimes couples break up during a pregnancy when new roles and responsibilities are not mutually acceptable or agreed on. In a study of lesbians' health concerns, Trippet and Bain (1990) reported that relationship issues were experienced by 77% of the women, followed by depression (65%), and conflict at work (63%). For example, one pregnant lesbian felt ambivalent about the attention she received at lesbian social gatherings, and complained to her partner about the group's raucous behavior. The couple's social network became a contention between them. Health care providers who are unfamiliar with lesbians' relationships and life-styles may fail to recognize maladaptive responses of the nonbiological parent that may jeopardize the pregnant partner (Wismont & Reame, 1989).

HOME VERSUS HOSPITAL CHILDBIRTH: DILEMMAS AND DECISIONS

Disenchantment with the patriarchal health care system and previous experiences of insensitivity to their life-styles have given lesbians justifiable reasons for seeking alternative health care providers. Fear of the unknown is paramount before and during the labor and delivery experience. In addition, stigmatization and ostracism by health care personnel are very real threats. Therefore, the fear of receiving less than optimal care, when they are extremely vulnerable to pain, loss of control, and death, is especially heightened for lesbians during childbirth (Wismont & Reame, 1989). Also, in the hospital setting, lesbian couples may not be allowed the same level of intimacy in language and comfort measures as heterosexual partners in labor (Wismont & Reame, 1989).

In Olesker and Walsh's (1984) study, 8 of the 9 lesbians chose midwives and sought out-of-hospital births. The vast majority of these women felt their midwives were supportive, and they were able to have friends from their lesbian community with them during childbirth. These women wanted a strong intrapartal female support system and drew from members of their lesbian community to provide that support. Their choice of out-of-hospital birth may have been tied to their desire for their friends' presence and support during childbirth, because most hospital only allow one support person at the birth. They also reported that they needed privacy and wanted to "be themselves" during the birthing experience. Five of these women felt this sense of privacy and comfort was not possible in a hospital setting. In choosing out-of-hospital birthing sites, laboring women may fear the need for emergency medical intervention and transport to a hospital during their labor.

In spite of their fears, Harvey et al. (1989) reported that more than 60% of the mothers in their study delivered in hospitals, 20% gave birth in out-of-hospital birthing centers, and 17% had home births. Lesbians in this study rated their comfort and satisfaction higher with midwives than with physicians. Those who delivered in hospitals may have preferred the availability of emergency equipment, accepted hospital delivery as the norm, or may not have had access to an acceptable provider who performed deliveries out of the hospital. Many lesbian couples have to compromise on the location of their delivery because of the limited options offered by their local health care providers.

EARLY MOTHERING/COPARENTING: DILEMMAS AND DECISIONS

During the first few weeks and months, both heterosexual and lesbian couples face many new changes and challenges. Whereas about 35% of all new mothers breastfeed their newborns, Harvey et al. (1989) found that 100% of the 35 lesbian mothers in their study breastfed their babies for at least 1 month, and 80% breastfed for 6 months or more. Although breastfeeding promotes a special bond between the mother and infant, the coparent may feel left out.

Lesbians view coparenting as different from the relationship of traditional couples, according to Olesker and Walsh (1984). Coparenting relationships were seen as more equal, with fewer power struggles between partners as compared with heterosexual marriages. However, "the ability of the nonchildbearing partner to formulate a parental role may be hindered by the feeling that she has no legal ties or obligations to the child" (Wismont & Reame, 1989, p. 138). The current law in many states makes adoption by the partner impossible, unless the biological mother gives up her rights to the child. Lesbian couples may fear that the grandparents' rights may take precedence over the nonbiological parent's right in a custody suit or that the social service system may have the power to remove the child from an "unfit" parent, whether biological or not. However, lesbian couples are still advised to establish contracts regarding the child's welfare in case of a separation or death of a partner.

Although commitment to children may provide a bond for most couples, the tentative nature of the lesbian relationship may create problems. The lack of state, family, or societal approval of lesbian unions may make it more difficult for couples to establish stable, strong, longlasting unions. Considering that a majority of lesbians already report relationship problems, depression, and conflict without children (Trippet & Bain, 1990), coparenting children may either add to their problems or provide a stronger bond.

Overcoming societal expectations that children live in a heterosexual home is a problem unique to lesbian families. Lesbian families may experience difficulty because of society's disapproval of raising children in homosexual families and the judicial system's reluctance to grant custody or allow adoption by same-sex partners. Lesbian parents must decide what (and when) to tell their child about his or her conception and life-style differences and how the child can explain the parents' life-style to classmates and friends.

Lesbian parents may also feel pulled in two directions. They may seek traditional mothers as role models to share their parenting experiences and concerns and for playmates for their children, yet may fear rejection and ostracism from these mothers if they disclose their sexual orientation. At the same time, lesbian parents usually hope to maintain their lesbian community of friends, but may be concerned about whether they will be accepted by nonmothers. Trying to find a comfortable balance and acceptance in both groups requires considerable effort.

Many biological lesbian mothers feel impelled to work to obtain health care insurance for themselves and their children. Because lesbian partners cannot be on each others' health insurance policies, and the nonbiological parent cannot have the child on her health plan, the biological parent cannot afford to be unemployed if she wants her child to receive the benefits and protection health insurance offers.

The nonbiological parent must contend with unique problems in the coparenting relationship. She often deals with the pressures of parenthood (sleepless nights and a sick baby) without any awareness or acknowledgment by coworkers of this major change in her life. Also, nonbiological parents are at the mercy of the biological parent: If the couple breaks up, they may worry about their future relationship with the child. Another concern of the nonbiological parent is what the child will call her—"mom," a first name, or what?

SUMMARY AND RECOMMENDATIONS

Lesbian childbearing couples are increasing in number and facing numerous decisions about how to conceive; where to give birth; which health care provider to choose; and how to cope with changes in their personal, family, and gay community relationships. Initially, each couple must face the potential effects of childbearing on their interpersonal relationship and their relationships within their supportive lesbian community. The benefits and risks of using donor insemination versus coitus, along with those of a known versus unknown donor, must also be considered. Selecting a sensitive health care provider who is accepting of their life-styles and supportive of their choice of birthing is another difficult decision for many lesbian couples. During pregnancy, lesbian couples usually attend childbirth education classes, but may feel isolated and uncomfortable. Normal physical and emotional changes during pregnancy may place strains on the couple's relationship, especially if the partner or the lesbian community is not as supportive of the pregnant lesbian as she expects. During childbirth, lesbian couples are especially vulnerable and have many fears of receiving inadequate care and possible harm in traditional health care institutions. Early coparenting experiences may be rewarding when the couple successfully negotiate their roles and the relationships between themselves, their families, and social networks. However, some lesbian coparents may receive no support from their families, friends, and health care providers and have difficulty establishing ties with heterosexual mothers. These couples may benefit from assistance in integrating an infant into their lives, balancing their relationship, and establishing a new network of friends. Lesbian childbearing couples will continue to struggle with each of these issues and concerns until society becomes more accepting of their life-styles.

Several recommendations have come from the few studies of lesbian childbearing couples available in the literature. Health care providers need to learn more about lesbians' life-styles and their health care concerns. Health care providers may acquire a better understanding of lesbians by reading traditional and underground literature and attending workshops that address the concerns of the gay and lesbian populations. Lesbians are looking for female providers who will avoid acting on the assumption that all women are heterosexual. They would like to be understood and accepted if they reveal their identity and not feel fearful that they might be rejected and possibly mistreated. Health care providers who adopt an open, sensitive, nonjudgmental attitude and are willing to listen to and respect lesbians as intelligent women with feelings will be sought out by this group.

Promoting lesbian health is a professional responsibility. Providing useful health care information in a meaningful, sensitive, and respectful way is very important. Maintaining confidentiality, including the partner in decision making, and asking questions in a sensitive manner are suggested strategies. Referring couples to lesbian mothers' support groups, if they are available, would be helpful. Ignoring their health care needs and withholding useful information may constitute negligent practice.

Further research into each of the phases of lesbians' childbearing experiences is needed. Because current research studies have sampled mainly white, middle-class, well-educated professionals, new studies should include lesbians representative of minority and diverse socioeconomic groups. As providers become better informed about and more receptive to the unique needs, desires, and expectations of childbearing lesbians, they will provide more appropriate assistance and support to these couples.

REFERENCES

Hall, M. (1978). Lesbian families. *Social Work, 23*, 380–385.

Harvey, S. M., Carr, C., & Bernheime, S. (1989). Lesbian mothers' health care experiences. *Jr. Nurse-Midwives, 34*(3), 115–119.

Hill, K. (1987). Mothers by insemination: Interviews. In S. Pollack & J. Vaughn (Eds.), *Politics of the heart: A lesbian parenting anthology* (pp. 111–119). Ithaca, NY: Firebrand Books.

Johnson, S. R., Smith, E. M., & Guenther, S. M. (1987). Parenting desires among bisexual women and lesbians. *Journal of Reproductive Medicine, 32*(3), 198–200.

Loulan, J. (1987). *Lesbian passion: Loving ourselves and each other.* San Francisco: Spinsters/Aunt Lute.

Murphy, M. (1987). And baby makes two. In S. Pollack & J. Vaughn (Eds.), *Politics of the heart: A lesbian anthology* (pp. 125–129). Ithaca, NY: Firebrand Books.

Olesker, E., & Walsh, L. V. (1984). Childbearing among lesbians: Are we meeting their needs? *Jr. Nurse-Midwives, 29*(5), 322–329.

Pollack, S. (1987). Lesbian mothers: A lesbian-feminist perspective on research. In S. Pollack, & J. Vaughn (Eds.), *Politics of the heart: A lesbian anthology* (pp. 316–324). Ithaca, NY: Firebrand Books.

Smith, E., Johnson, S., & Guenther, S. (1985). Health care attitudes and experiences during gynecologic care among lesbians and bisexuals. *American Journal of Public Health, 75*, 1085–1987.

Stevens, P. E., & Hall, J. M. (1988). Stigma, health beliefs, and experiences with health care in lesbian women. *Image: Journal of Nursing Scholarship, 20*(2), 69–73.

Tolor, A., & Degrazia, P. (1976). Sexual attitudes and behavior patterns during and following pregnancy. *Archives of Sexual Behavior, 5*, 539–551.

Trippet, S., & Bain, J. (1990). Preliminary study of lesbian health concerns. *Health Values, 14*(6), 30–36.

Van Gelder, L. (1991). A lesbian family revisited. *MS., 1*(5), 44–47.

Wismont, J. M., & Reame, N. E. (1989). The lesbian childbearing experience: Assessing development tasks. *Image: Journal of Nursing Scholarship, 21*(3), 137–141.

Zook, N., & Hallenback, R. (1987). Lesbian co-parenting: Creating connections. In S. Pollack & J. Vaughn (Eds.), *Politics of the heart: A lesbian anthology* (pp. 89–93). Ithaca, NY: Firebrand Books.

AN INVESTIGATION OF THE HEALTH CARE PREFERENCES OF THE LESBIAN POPULATION

Vicki A. Lucas, RNC, PhD

Memorial Hospital Southwest, Houston, Texas

A descriptive study was done to explore the health care preferences of 178 self-identified lesbians. They were surveyed regarding their preferences for health care services, health care providers, clinic logistics, and identification and documentation of sexual preference. Holistic counseling, health maintenance, and disease prevention services were identified as their top priorities. Female health care providers were identified as a priority, and most of the women felt that sexual preference should be asked but not recorded in the chart.

In this article I report the findings of a study that I conducted to explore the health care preferences of the lesbian community. The intent of the study was to ascertain the types of health care services that lesbians desired, the type of health care environment they preferred, the type of health care providers they preferred, and their preferences regarding the asking and recording of sexual preference.

Numerous investigators have demonstrated that lesbians avoid or delay seeking care because of the insensitivity of health care personnel and because of how poorly the medical system has related to their sexual preference (Johnson, Guenther, Laube, & Keettel, 1981; Malterud, 1986; Raymond, 1988; Smith, Johnson, & Guenther, 1985; Stevens & Hall, 1988; Zeidenstein, 1991). These same studies have also documented that lesbians believe that disclosure of their sexual preference to their physicians would negatively affect the quality of health care they would receive, and some even believe they would risk harm in some health care situations. The assumption of heterosexuality, which is pervasive within the medical system, is offensive to lesbians and has re-

I acknowledge the assistance of Julie Richards, RNC, MSN, and Harriett Linenberger, RNC, MSN, with data collection.

sulted in negative experiences for lesbians within that system. This as
sumption is so embedded within the system that most lesbians report
never being asked their sexual preference (Johnson et al., 1981; Smith et
al., 1985; Stevens & Hall, 1988; Zeidenstein, 1991).

Numerous writers speak to the health care needs and preferences of
gay males and heterosexual females, yet lesbians are all but ignored.
The limited knowledge about the health care needs of the lesbian population as well as their delay in seeking health care have profound implications for their health status.

METHOD

In this descriptive study I explored the health care preferences of the
lesbian population in a large city in the southwestern United States. A
survey was constructed to obtain information on health care needs as
well as health care preferences within the lesbian community. The
results of the survey were used to develop lesbian health care services
within a gay-community-based health care clinic.

Sample

The convenience sample comprised 178 self-identified lesbian
women. They ranged in age from 18 to 55 years, with a mean age of 28.
Their income ranged from $8,000 to $60,000, with a median of
$26,000. Ninety percent of the sample was employed, 1% was unem-
ployed, and 9% were full-time students. The range of jobs was from
waitress to physician, with the majority of the sample employed in semi-
professional jobs (see Table 1 for additional demographic characteristics
of the sample).

Procedure

A questionnaire was developed by the investigator and was used to
explore health care preferences of lesbians. The questionnaire was analyzed for content validity by a panel of experts. The questionnaire was
pilot tested at a lesbian support group meeting to assess clarity, ease of
administration, and accuracy of information.

Questionnaires were distributed in various places where the lesbian
population could be located. Leaders within the lesbian community as-
sisted with data collection and with communications about the survey.
Data were collected at lesbian support groups, lesbian social clubs, athletic events, and gay coalition functions. Data were analyzed using descriptive statistics.

Table 1. Demographic Characteristics of the Women in the Sample

	Sample	
Variable	n	%
Race		
White	171	85
Hispanic	18	10
Black	5	3
Oriental	4	2
Highest level of education		
Graduate degree	9	5
Baccalaureate degree	103	58
Associate degree	21	12
Trade school	27	15
High school	16	9
Less than high school	2	1
Primary relationship status		
Living with partner	65	37
Date one partner	82	40
Divorced	11	6
Legally married	11	6
Single	5	3
Multiple partners	4	2

RESULTS

Health Care Services

The women in the sample were asked to identify and prioritize the health care services they would use. Table 2 lists the services identified by the women in order of priority. Services that were not selected by any of the women were prenatal care, mammography, sex preselection, parenting classes, childbirth education classes, postpartum care, and alcohol/drug abuse counseling. When asked if they would use the clinic for their primary health care needs, 44% of the women indicated they would, 41% indicated they were undecided, and 15% indicated they would not.

Health Care Environment

The women were then asked to respond to the statement "I would prefer to attend the clinic during designated hours specifically for women." The results of this item can be found in Table 3.

Table 2. Priority List of Health Care Services Identified

Service	Frequency (% of total sample)
Pap smear	87.9
Breast examination	66.7
Pelvic examination	57.6
Well-woman health classes	54.6
Vaginitis treatment	48.5
General physical examination	42.4
Psychological counseling	42.4
Nutrition counseling	36.4
Exercise counseling	36.4
Sexuality counseling	33.3
Premenstrual stress management	33.3
Spiritual counseling	33.3
Sexually transmitted diseases screening	33.3
Eating disorders treatment	30.3
Human immunodeficiency virus (HIV) screening	24.2
Benign breast disease management	24.2
Uterine bleeding management	21.2
Artificial insemination	18.8
Menopause management	15.2
HIV counseling	9.3
Abuse/battering counseling	9.1
Pregnancy confirmation	6.1
Pregnancy counseling	3.0

Table 3. Preference for Clinic Hours Designated Specifically for Women

Preference	Frequency (%)
Strongly agree	30.3
Agree	27.3
Neutral	24.2
Disagree	18.2
Strong disagree	0

Two subsequent items asked the women what days of the week and hours of the day they prefer services to be available. Fifty percent of the women chose Saturday, 20% chose Sunday, and 30% chose Monday. Approximately 70% of the women chose 6:00 P.M. to 10:00 P.M. as the most convenient hours for services.

Health Care Providers

The women were asked to identify and prioritize the types of health care personnel they prefer. The results of this item can be found in Table 4. It is not surprising that 92% of the women indicated a preference for a lesbian health care provider.

Sexual Preference

In the last two items on the survey, the women were asked if sexual preference should be asked routinely on a health history and if sexual preference should be recorded on the chart. Table 5 shows their responses.

DISCUSSION

The women clearly identified cancer screening and detection and well-woman care as the top-priority health care services they desired.

Table 4. Priority List of Health Care Providers Identified

Personnel	Frequency (% of total sample)
Female family practice physician	78.1
Female nurse practitioner	71.9
Female OB/GYN physician	65.6
Female physician assistant	56.3
Female nurse midwife	43.8
Female volunteers	43.8
Male nurse practitioner	15.6
Male physician assistant	15.6
Male volunteers	15.6
Male OB/GYN physician	12.5
Male family practice physician	12.5
Male nurse midwife	9.4

**Table 5. Preference for Asking Sexual Preference and
Recording Preference on the Chart**

Preference	Ask sexual preference (%)	Record on chart (%)
Strongly agree	33.3	6.3
Agree	30.3	21.9
Neutral	12.1	15.6
Disagree	3.0	15.6
Strongly disagree	21.2	40.6

Lesbians have been found to have a slightly higher risk for the delayed detection of cervical dysplasia. Also, they may be at increased risk for breast and endometrial cancer due to their high incidence of nulliparity. Health education and counseling of various types were identified as second in priority by the women. There is an increased rate of depression, suicide, anxiety, and psychological treatment among lesbians. The women identified treatment of minor health deviations as third in priority, with the exception of the treatment of vaginitis, which ranked higher. This is consistent with studies that have identified vaginitis as the most common health problem among lesbians.

It is of interest that screening for sexually transmitted diseases ranked in the bottom third of the women's priorities. This is consistent with studies that have found that lesbians have one of the lowest rates of sexually transmitted diseases. Human immunodeficiency virus (HIV) screening and counseling were ranked in the lower third of priorities by the women. It is of interest that it was listed as a priority at all because lesbians constitute one of the lowest risk populations for contracting HIV. The explanations for this priority may be their previous IV drug use, heterosexual exposure, or use of unscreened male homosexual semen for artificial insemination.

Respondents' identification of the need for sexual assault counseling is consistent with the studies that found that many lesbians have been victims of incest or sexual assault. The identified need for abuse/battering counseling is also consistent with studies that have documented domestic violence as a problem among lesbians. The low ranking of menopause management may be related to the young age of the women. I was surprised at the low or absent interest in pregnancy-related services. There appears to be a baby boom among the lesbian community, but these women identified obstetrical services as a low priority. The exclusion of alcohol/drug abuse counseling is inconsistent with studies that have documented an increased incidence of alcoholism and drug addiction in the lesbian population. Also, the exclusion of mammography is inconsistent with the identification of cancer screening and detection as a high priority. Possibly, mammography may be perceived as exploitive medical technology, or the exclusion may be related to the relatively young age of the women.

Clearly the preference for clinic days and hours is reflective of the high employment rate of the women. However, the lack of consensus on hours designated for women only is somewhat surprising given the assumption that lesbians would be more comfortable in a setting with only female clients.

The overwhelming preference for female health care providers and for lesbian providers is consistent with the findings of many studies. It is of interest that the women ranked family practice physicians above OB/GYN physicians. This may be related to the negative experiences that many lesbians have had with OB/GYN physicians or lesbians' perception of a need for a broader based form of care. Also, the women ranked the female nurse practitioner above the female OB/GYN physician.

The majority (63%) of the women felt that sexual preference should be asked in a health history, but only 28% felt that this information should be recorded on the chart. In fact, half the women (50%) felt that sexual preference should not be included on the record. This is consistent with studies that have documented that most lesbians would prefer to be asked their sexual preference but prefer that information to be kept confidential between themselves and their health care providers.

CONCLUSION

A descriptive study of 178 lesbians was undertaken to identify the health care preferences of the lesbian population. The women identified 24 health care services that they desired. Cancer screening and detection, health education, and holistic counseling were identified as the priority health care services desired. Screening and management of minor health deviations were listed as lower priorities. One can extrapolate from these priorities that lesbians perceive health care as health oriented, not medicine or cure oriented. The women prioritized their preferences for various types of health care providers. Females, preferably lesbians, were a higher priority than males, and in several cases nonphysician providers were preferred over physicians, especially OB/GYN physicians. Last, lesbians preferred to have sexual preference asked in a health history but did not feel this information should be recorded on the chart.

Numerous investigators have estimated that 2–6% of the female population is exclusively homosexual and that 20% of all women have some lesbian contact before the age of 40. They have suggested also that lesbians are dissatisfied with the present health care delivery system and avoid using it. Lesbians are an overlooked and underserved population whose health care needs are unique and must be met. If they are to have a positive impact on the health status of the lesbian population, health care providers and educators need to incorporate the information from this research into their practice and teaching.

REFERENCES

Johnson, S. R., Guenther, S. M., Laube, D. W., & Keettel, W. C. (1981). Factors influencing lesbian gynecologic care: A preliminary study. *American Journal of Obstetrics and Gynecology, 140,* 20–28.

Malterud, K. (1986). Health matters in lesbian women. *Tidsskr. Nor Laegeforen, 106,* 2071–2074.

Raymond, C. A. (1988). Lesbians call for greater physician awareness, sensitivity to improve patient care. *Journal of the American Medical Association, 259,* 18.

Smith, E. M., Johnson, S. R., & Guenther, S. M. (1985). Health care attitudes and experiences during gynecologic care among lesbians and bisexuals. *American Journal of Public Health, 75,* 1085–1087.

Stevens, P. E., & Hall, J. M. (1988). Stigma, health beliefs, and experiences with health care in lesbian women. *Image: Journal of Nursing Scholarship, 20*(2), 69–73.

Zeidenstein, L. (1991). Gynecological and childbearing needs of lesbians. *Journal of Nurse-Midwifery, 35*(1), 10–18.

THE LESBIAN CUSTODY PROJECT

Jill Radford

Rights of Women, London, United Kingdom

In the United Kingdom the backlash against feminism in the late 1980s was initially directed at lesbians and was specifically focused on lesbians who are mothers, lesbians engaged in parenting, or lesbians wishing to do so. This backlash was initially orchestrated by a small group of far right politicians, well to the right of the Thatcher government, and was not contained in any political consensus but was developed into a major public issue by the media. This paper documents its effect in terms of a systematic legal attack on lesbian parenting. The aim of the paper is to alert readers to the backlash with a view to resistance. Our argument is that the backlash against lesbians is a first line of attack against all women as mothers.

NEWS FROM THE UNITED KINGDOM: BACKLASH AGAINST LESBIAN PARENTING— FIRST IT WAS CLAUSE 28 AND THEN . . .

As the Lesbian Custody Project* documented in its *Lesbian Mothers' Legal Handbook* (Lesbian Custody Group, Rights of Women, 1986), lesbians have never exactly been the flavor of the month when it comes to parenting or child care issues. Whether a lesbian has children as a consequence of marriage or a heterosexual relationship or through insemination, she may face a legal dispute with the child's father over who should bring up the child (i.e., custody) and what contact the other parent should have with the child (i.e., access). She will certainly face widespread hostility and discrimination as a lesbian mother. Given that

---

*The Lesbian Custody Project is a project based at Rights of Women, in London. It was started in 1982 to support lesbian mothers involved in contested custody disputes regarding their children. Recently, responding to the events described in this article, we have expanded our work to include all aspects of lesbian parenting.

139

the legal system in Great Britain is also characterized by racism and is biased in favor of the middle classes, a lesbian mother from a minority ethnic background who is working class will additionally have to deal with the law's race and class biases. Similarly, a lesbian mother with disabilities will have to face the dominant assumption that an ideal mother is fully able bodied. Thus the hostility faced by a lesbian mother may be compounded by other forms of discrimination, depending on her background.

In custody disputes, the lesbian's parenting abilities and material circumstances and the child(ren)'s wishes take second place to an investigation of her personal relationships, politics, and sexuality. She may be subjected to personal abuse or insult from Court Welfare officers, the father, his lawyers, and even the judge and will certainly feel put on trial.

One result of publication of the Lesbian Custody Project's handbook and the training work it has engaged in with lawyers, social workers, and students of these professions is that mothers have been better prepared, better advised, and better represented, to the extent that although a custody dispute is still hard to fight and remains an ordeal, the result is no longer a foregone conclusion and lesbian mothers have quietly begun to win some cases.

THE CLAUSE

However, just about when it might have been noticed that we were making some progress in our struggle to create a situation in which lesbian mothers were treated by the courts in the same way as our heterosexual sisters, we were faced with Section 2A* of the Local Government Act of 1988. This section represented a fundamental attack on the civil rights of the lesbian and gay communities as a whole, but specifically affected lesbian mothers and their children by naming us "pretended family relationships."

---

*Section 2A of the Local Government Act of 1988 reads,

  (1) A local authority shall not:
     a) intentionally promote homosexuality or publish material with the intention of promoting homosexuality;
     b) promote the teaching in any maintained school of the acceptability of homosexuality as a pretended family relationship. (Colvin & Hawksley, 1989, p. 65)

Throughout the passage of this act through Parliament, this section, initially known as Clause 28 and later as Section 28, was the target of much criticism and activism, from the lesbian and

DONOR INSEMINATION

The attack on lesbian parenting did not stop with Section 28. It surfaced again in the debate around the Human Embryology and Fertilisation Bill in 1989. The first evidence we had that something nasty was going on was the Early Day Motion of October 26, 1989 ("Early Day Motion," 1990). This pernicious motion, signed by Members of Parliament (MPs)—Ann Winterton, Jill Knight, and David Wiltshire among others—was completely unambiguous:

> That this House notes with profound concern the recent revelation that 55 lesbian couples and eight single lesbians have been impregnated by one sperm bank alone during the last three years; expresses its dismay at the ease with which these and two thousand other unmarried women who are not infertile were able to gain access to such facilities; believes that such practices undermine the status of marriage, corrupt the family unit, and leave the ensuing children at grave risk of emotional harm; and calls upon the Secretary of State to review his policy on such matters and to bring forward legislation before the House which will enable it to come to a decision as to whether or not such practices should be allowed. (Early Day Motion, no. 1324, Hansard Order Paper no. 165.)

THE HUMAN EMBRYOLOGY AND FERTILISATION BILL

Unfortunately, the supporters of this motion had their wish. The Human Embryology and Fertilisation Bill of 1989/1990 proved to be opportune. This bill, which was concerned primarily with new reproductive technologies, was in part hijacked by those wishing to deny lesbians and single women access to a much older technology, donor insemination. The first attempt to do this occurred in the House of Lords with amendments made by Lady Saltoun of Abernathy that attempted to outlaw in vitro fertilization for unmarried women and to provide that in no circumstances can a license authorize any treatment

---

gay communities in the United Kingdom. These campaigns attracted support from lesbians and gays throughout the European Community. The campaigns targeted the entire section, which was recognized as a fundamental attack on the already very limited civil rights of lesbians and gay men. Of particular concern to lesbian mothers was its specific attack on us and our children in the phrase "pretended family relationship." Although this legislation has no direct bearing on decisions in the family court, because it is local government legislation, it clearly affects the political climate in which decisions in family law are reached.

services (e.g., donor insemination) to unmarried women.* Though expressed in terms of unmarried women, this represented an explicit attack on the rights of lesbians and single women, in keeping with the Early Day Motion. Interestingly, this law allows single women to be treated less favorably than married women, but not the reverse. Nevertheless, this amendment was defeated in the House of Lords, but by only one vote.

The site of struggle then shifted to the House of Commons. There attention was primarily focused on other amendments aimed at further reducing abortion rights. These were lost after heated debate in the full chamber of the House, and all other measures were debated in committee.

In committee, MPs Jill Knight, Ann Winterton, and David Wiltshire introduced a series of amendments aimed at denying donor insemination to single women and lesbians. Because they could not reintroduce amendments thrown out by the House of Lords, each attempt was worded differently. At one point they even tried one that stated that a woman could not have access to these services unless she was accompanied by a man. These were defeated in committee, arousing the ire of even some Tory MPs like Edwina Curry, who raised the specter of women picking up men at bus stops to take to the clinic and the situation of women whose husbands drop dead on the steps of the clinic.

Aided by briefing papers from the Lesbian Custody Project and the Campaign for Access to Donor Insemination (CADI), a campaign group established around this as a single issue, these measures were rejected in committee, presumably as too crude and obvious in the state's attempt to control women's fertility. Even Virginia Bottomley, then Minister of Health, was opposed to such obviously oppressive measures, arguing that the trio's concerns were already met by the incorporation of a statement of the welfare principle in the bill.

At this point the bill was returned to the full House for its last reading. However, the dissatisfied trio made a further and successful attempt to restrict fertility services to married or "stable cohabiting heterosexual couples," with a majority of 52 votes accepting David Wiltshire's last-minute amendment to the welfare principle. The restated welfare principle now reads:

---

*In vitro fertilization is a highly technical procedure, in which a woman is caused to superovulate (producing an average of seven or eight eggs in one cycle) by the use of fertility drugs. The eggs produced are then removed surgically, fertilized with sperm in a laboratory, and if judged to be healthy the resulting embryos are placed in the woman's womb.

A woman shall not be provided with treatment services unless account has been taken of the welfare of any child who may be born as a result of the treatment, and of any other child who may be affected by the birth, including the need of that child for a father. ("Human Embryology and Fertilisation Bill," 1990, p. 4879)

Although supporters of this amended welfare principle may be reluctant to admit it publicly, their concern, as the Early Day Motion illustrated, is clearly to prevent lesbians from using clinics.

In this way, the act as passed by the House of Commons has serious implications for all single women seeking donor insemination from a clinic. It will affect lesbians particularly. It was argued by the government that the new law brings donor insemination in line with other child care legislation that is based on the welfare principle.

THE WELFARE PRINCIPLE

The history of the welfare principle in family law dates back to the 1886 Guardianship of Infants Act. This act challenged paternal rights by allowing mothers, after a divorce, to claim custody of their child(ren) up to the age of 21 years. Previously, mothers could only be granted custody until a child was 7. However, the act also directed the courts for the first time to have regard for the welfare of the child in making decisions around custody and access. The welfare principle was strengthened in the 1925 Guardianship of Infants Act, which established that the child's welfare was the first and paramount consideration in custody disputes, rather than the competing claims of the parents. No one would argue with the principle of prioritizing a child's welfare, but in practice what this has meant historically in the English legal system is that the patriarchal state, as represented by judges, is given absolute discretion to decide what is in the child's best interests and thereby to define the idealized role of motherhood.

In the context of the Human Embryology and Fertilisation Bill, this means that certain women will be considered fit to conceive a child and others will not. Clinics that provide donor insemination will be asked to evaluate not the actual parenting abilities of a woman, but her potential parenting abilities. They will be considering not the welfare of an actual child, but that of a potential child. It is unclear what if any criteria would be appropriate in this situation or how any assessment can be undertaken. In the absence of any clear criteria, presumably any such judgments will fall back on the idealized white, heterosexual, ablebodied, middle-class family norm, and thus women outside this "persil family" model will be discriminated against.

The Code of Practice published in March 1991 emphasizes that clinics will be bound by law to "take account of the need of *that* child for a father" but qualifies this as follows:

> Where the child will have no legal father, centers are required to have regard to that child's need for a father and should pay particular attention to the prospective mother's ability to meet the child's needs throughout his or her childhood. ("Human Embryology and Fertilisation Act," 1991)

It should be noted, however, that the act refers to *that* child, rather than *the* child. As the Code of Practice implies, it is therefore quite possible for a sympathetic clinic to look at the woman's particular circumstances and conclude that her child has no particular need for a father and that the mother has the ability to provide for the needs of the child. However, the law is bound to deter those clinics with doubts from providing donor insemination to lesbians and women without male partners.

Although the practical consequences of this law must be small, because such treatments are highly expensive and accorded low priority in our overextended National Health Service, its ideological impact cannot be underestimated. The welfare clause needs to be seen in the context of other policy attempts to bolster the heterosexual "persil" family as the normal and only acceptable context for children.

The apparent threat to men or family life posed by fertile women seeking donor insemination reached the state of hysteria in the press when, in March 1991, a news story was constructed on the theme of "virgin birth," referring to the fact that a single woman who had never had heterosexual intercourse was receiving donor insemination treatment. Presented in the press as a threat to family life and society as we know it, the fear of male redundancy reached dramatic proportions. At the Lesbian Custody Project, we were inundated by requests for statements on virgin births, which was seen as something new and highly alarming, although presumably self-insemination is as old as heterosexuality itself, and certainly is not new technology. Although under pressure to change the law, the government is currently standing by the wording of the 1990 Human Embryology and Fertilisation Act, and veiled threats have been made that clinics acting out of line are in danger of losing their licenses to practice.

LESBIAN FOSTERING AND ADOPTION

The ink was hardly dry on the Human Embryology and Fertilisation Act when lesbian parenting was once again the subject of a hysterical attack and moral panic. After a press campaign attacking social service departments in London and around the country for allowing lesbians to become foster and adoptive parents, there was yet another Early Day Motion. This one read,

> That this house unreservedly condemns the actions of Newcastle City Council in removing a handicapped boy from his foster mother to be adopted by a lesbian couple; utterly rejects the abhorrent claim by the City Council that the decision is in the best interests of the child; reaffirms the position of the traditional family unit as the most secure and stable means of raising all children, especially the most impressionable and vulnerable; and believes that the placing of young children with lesbian couples is not suitable to the needs or best interests of these children and despite the protestations of the homosexual lobby, never will be. (25 Oct. 1990, Hansard no. 1429, p. 4879)

Newcastle City Council was forced to take out an injunction to end the sensationalist press reports of the particular case, so it cannot be discussed here.

In and of itself, an Early Day Motion does not amount to more than an MP's petition. However, what usually happens when there is support for an Early Day Motion is that its proponents attempt to incorporate it, by tabling an amendment, into the first convenient bill. This is how both the infamous Section 28 and now the antilesbian amendment to the Human Embryology and Fertilisation Act started their Parliamentary lives.

LESBIAN CUSTODY: RECENT DECISIONS

These last few months, then, have seen a mounting of a systematic attack on lesbian parenting. In this context, the Lesbian Custody Project was pleasantly surprised by the recent outcomes of two contested custody hearings. In both, care and control were awarded to the lesbian mother, despite the intervention of the Appeal Court in one of them ("Nearest the Norm," 1990). In this case, the father appealed against the judge's decision to award care and control of a 7-year-old girl to her lesbian mother. At the first hearing, the judge ruled that each parent could offer the same standard of child care and reasonable access to the other parent. Whether she lived with her mother or her father, the judge argued, the child would have to cope with her mother's lesbian relationship. So given the close bond between mother and daughter, it would be in her best interests to be with her mother.

The Appeal Court disagreed. Lords Justice Glidewell and Balcombe argued that when the court had to decide which of two households best met the needs of the child, it had to choose that nearest to the idealized persil family norm, or as they put it, "the one closest to the ideal represented by a harmonious matrimonial environment" (Glidewell &

Balcombe, 1990, p. 23). The Appeal Court judges went on to articulate the standard myths about how a lesbian relationship was an unusual background for a child, though Lord Glidewell was careful to say that being in a lesbian relationship did not conclusively disqualify a mother from having care and control: "A court might well decide that such a sensitive, loving relationship was a more satisfactory environment for a child than the alternative, but the nature of the relationship was important and should be put into a balance" (Glidewell & Balcombe, 1990, p. 23).

They then ordered that the mother and father should have joint custody but ordered a rehearing before the Family Division of the High Court to decide care and control. The story thus far was well aired in the national press. What was given less publicity was the fact that after a 3-day hearing, Justice Booth gave unconditional care and control to the mother.

THE PRESS

As always, the negativity of the Appeal Court was well publicized, but the fact that the proceedings concluded with the child's being returned to her mother was kept much quieter. It is this selective reporting by the press that gives judges the impression that it is unusual, and therefore in some way problematic, for a child to live with his or her lesbian mother. This silence around lesbian mothering allows the press to engage in sensationalist reporting and the generation of moral panics. These then can feed into the political discourse and produce antilesbian legislation, as has been outlined here. For lesbian mothers the selective reporting of antilesbian decisions is dangerous because it may lead to their thinking they stand no chance in court. This is not currently the case. Lesbian custody cases are hard to fight, and the backlash does not help. But despite the discrimination against lesbian mothers, the stress and anxiety involved in contesting cases, and the experience of being put on trial in court, the Lesbian Custody Project is finding that it is possible still to win individual cases.

REFERENCES

Colvin, Madeleine, & Hawksley, Jane. 1989. *Section 28: A practical guide to the law and its implications.* London: Liberty.
Early Day Motion no. 1324. 1989, October 25. Impregnation of Lesbian Women. *Hansard Order Paper no. 165*, 1 November 1989, no. 6211. Ref. H 5309.
Glidewell & Balcome. (1990, November). *Family Law Journal*, p. 23.

Human Fertility and Embryology Act. (1991, March). *Code of Practice. Consultation Document*.

Human Embryology and Fertilisation Bill, No. 1429. (1990, October 25). *Hansard*, p. 4879.

Lesbian Custody Group, Rights of Women. (1986). *Lesbian mothers legal handbook*. London: Women's Press.

Nearest the norm. (1990). *Family Law, 20,* 413–414.

INDEX

Acquired immune deficiency syndrome (*see* AIDS)
AIDS, 47, 50, 122
Alcohol abuse, 109–110
    as coping mechanism, 110, 113, 115, 116
    Deevey-Wall model, 113–117
    Finnegan-McNally model, 110–113
Alcohol problems, 91–94
    images of recovery, 95–96
        as connection/reconnection, 99–100
        as cyclical/celebratry, 100
        as empowerment, 102
        as personal growth, 96–97
        as physical transition, 96
        as reclaiming the self, 98
        as social transition, 102–103
        as struggle with compulsivity, 97–98
        as vocational change, 101
    implications for health care, 103–106
        abuse survivors, 105
        incest, 105
    recovery from, 93–94
Alternative health care practices, 56, 120
American Psychological Association, 42, 84
Artificial insemination, 87–88, 122
    (*See also* Conception)
Assumption of heterosexuality, 66, 69
At-risk population, 109
Attitudes toward lesbians, (table) 3–6, 18–19

Bem Sex Role Inventory, 45
Blaming the victim, 42
Breast cancer, 136

Campaign for Access to Donor Insemination (CADI), UK, 142
Cervical dysplasia, 136
Childbearing plans, 76
Childbearing process, 119
Coming out, 31–32, 35, 69–70, 85
    confidentiality, 85
    discrimination:
        employment, 86
        housing, 86
    gay-bashing, 86
    humiliation, 185
    rejection, 85
    shame, 85

Conception, 121–123
    AIDS, 122
    artificial insemination, 122
Coparenting, 126–127
    adoption, 126
        (*See also* Lesbian adoption)
    depression, 126

Deevey-Wall model, 113–117
Delayed help seeking, 23–24
Disclosure of identity, 21–23
Discrimination:
    employment, 86
    housing, 86
    seeking health care and, 71
Donor insemination, UK, 141

Early mothering, 126–127
Ecological transition, 33–35
    consequences, of coming out, 35
    extension of knowledge, 36
    framework for intervention, 36–37
    implications for health care providers:
        negative attitudes of self, 37–38
        negative attitudes of students, 41
    social stigma, 37
Endometrial cancer, 136

Fear of seduction, 48–49
Feminist theory, 55–56
Financial support, 26–27
Finnegan-McNally model, 110–113

Gay bar, 110
Gay-bashing, 86
Gynecological health care, 119
Gynecological and obstetrical problems, 56

Health care experiences, (table) 7–17, 19, 24–25
    antipathy, 19–21
    delayed help seeking, 23
    disclosure of identity, 21
    financial support, 26–27
    ignorance, 19–21
    knowledge development, 25–26
    research development, 25–26

T - #0576 - 101024 - C0 - 212/152/9 - PB - 9781560322993 - Gloss Lamination